How to Beat

Insomnia and Sleep Problems

One Step at a Time

D1245576

How to Beat

Insomnia and Sleep Problems

One Step at a Time

Kirstie Anderson

ROBINSON

ROBINSON

First published in Great Britain in 2018 by Robinson

1 3 5 7 9 10 8 6 4 2

Important Note
This book is not intended as a substitute for medical advice
or treatment. Any person with a condition requiring medical
attention should consult a qualified medical practitioner or
suitable therapist.

A CIP catalogue record for this book
is available from the British Library.

ISBN: 978-1-47214-058-6

Typeset in Minion by Initial Typesetting Services, Edinburgh
Printed and bound in Great Britain by Clays Ltd, Elcograf S.p.A.

Papers used by Robinson are from well-managed forests and other
responsible sources.

MIX
Paper from
responsible sources
FSC® C104740

Robinson
An imprint of
Little, Brown Book Group
Carmelite House
50 Victoria Embankment
London EC4Y 0DZ

An Hachette UK Company
www.hachette.co.uk

www.littlebrown.co.uk

CONTENTS

Section 1: Getting going   1

Section 2: Understanding sleep: how and
    why we do it, and why does it go wrong   21

Section 3: Techniques to improve your sleep   57

    Week 1 – Assessing and measuring your sleep   58

    Week 2 – Sleep hygiene and relaxation   65

    Week 3 – Sleep scheduling   76

    Week 4 – Adjusting the sleep schedule   91

    Week 5 – How to slow down a racing mind
       and fall asleep more easily   96

    Week 6 – Putting it all together and
       keeping it together   105

Section 4: Recovery stories   115

Resources   145

Index   166

Section 1

GETTING GOING

Good to meet you!

I am sorry that you are struggling to sleep well; this can be incredibly frustrating, but I am really glad that you have started reading this book. I hope that you find it helpful. It is designed to teach you more about your sleep and to help you sleep better at night if you are struggling with insomnia. Many people sleep badly, sometimes for years. They feel that this really affects their mood and performance the next day. However, I want to try and give you a toolkit with techniques you can use for better nights and therefore better days. I have tried to put as much useful information about sleep into the book as possible.

The techniques I will teach you are based upon Cognitive Behavioural Therapy (CBT) specifically for insomnia. You may have heard about CBT. This is a psychological or 'talking therapy', which is often used to treat other problems such as anxiety or depression. However, I know that your problem is very much around sleep itself. So, our main focus will be on the night and the bedroom.

The book is broken down into sections that explain sleep: what it is and how it works. Then there are short sections that help you to understand your sleep and give you a six-week plan to improve your insomnia. I will also introduce you to other people who have worked through the techniques themselves, what worked for them, whether some parts were tougher than others and how they felt as things improved over time. I will break down each step for you and, at times, each hour of the night. The book will help you work through these steps week by week, first to measure your own sleep and then put the techniques in place to improve it. There is also lots of extra information and resources at the end of the book that many of my patients have found to be helpful.

About myself

I should introduce myself, explain a bit about who I am and why I have written this book. I'm a consultant neurologist within the Newcastle Regional Sleep Service and an honorary senior lecturer at Newcastle University. I see and treat people with all kinds of sleep disorders. So I listen to bedtime stories for a living!

About fifteen years ago, I first found out about CBT for insomnia (CBTi) and started to use these techniques with the patients who came to see me with this problem. They worked so well, even for those who had slept badly for years, that I wanted far more people to know about CBTi. I now work in one of the biggest Sleep Services in the country within a large team. We are all passionate about helping our patients to get a good night's sleep. Many of us see and treat patients with insomnia. I run annual training courses for other health professionals teaching them about sleep and insomnia. I have designed online treatment programmes that are now available within the NHS and have developed training materials for the latest national programme of talking therapy services in England.

My research interests are around the role that sleep disturbance has in mental health problems. Given how vital good sleep is for normal memory and mood, I work closely with psychiatrists to understand and improve bad sleep in those with mental health problems. My home interests are running around muddy cross-country fields and adapting to the long lie-ins of my teenage children.

So what is CBTi (Cognitive Behavioural Therapy for insomnia)?

The techniques in this book are based on many years of careful research work on literally thousands of patients with severe insomnia. This is a clinically proven and effective treatment, and it is recommended by the National Institute for Health and Care Excellence (NICE) who provide national guidance on the best available treatments. CBTi techniques are shown to be either as effective or more effective than other treatments such as sleeping pills (of which more later). One issue has been a lack of awareness about CBTi therapy, which may be why you have not tried it before.

These techniques have been shown to be effective when used face-to-face with a therapist, but also in groups or using computerised versions of the therapy. In other words, however we teach you these techniques, they seem to work for most people.

Using this book

You are best to think of this book as a course of treatment; I have tried to write it with this in mind. If you have not used any form of self-help book before or considered CBT, this may seem a little daunting, particularly if you already feel that your thinking isn't as clear as it should be after a bad night! However, I have broken the book down into short sections to let you work through it at a pace that suits you. So this is a manual – giving you a '**what** to do', and 'exactly **how** to do it'.

Your doctor or counsellor may have recommended this book and, if so, you can work through it together. If you are working through it on your own, then you may want to highlight helpful bits as you go along. Please write in this book! For lots of us, writing in books is something we were always told not to do. For a self-help book you have to break this rule because generally the more writing you do the better. CBTi works best when people complete the treatment programme as it is laid out week by week and over a six- to seven-week period.

There are four sections in the book; the first two tell you how to get going and give you lots of information about your sleep to turn you into your own sleep expert. Section 3 contains the sleep treatment programme. Section 4 tells you about Paul and Poppy who both had bad sleep but recovered. At the back of the book, there are lots of resources and extra information to support you as well as the weekly sleep diaries you will need during treatment.

Section 1: Getting going

Here I will try to help you to understand why this treatment might work for you even if other things that you have tried have failed. I'll explain how to approach the therapy and when it is best for you to start. Also, I will give you some simple tips to increase your chances of success.

Section 2: Understanding sleep

This is vital and really interesting for most of us – good and bad sleepers alike. There is surprisingly little knowledge about sleep among healthcare professionals, considering that we spend about one third of our lives asleep. So, I will explain how we measure sleep (there is lots of detail in the back of the book as well), how it changes over time and then how insomnia and poor sleep develops. Recognising other common sleep disorders is also important. Bad sleep can have several causes, so we will cover this as well. Some people have taken sleeping tablets in the past or are taking them now, and I will explain how this therapy can fit in with other treatment you may be on.

By the end of this section you will have covered much of the information I teach to those who come to our training courses to learn about sleep medicine. I want to help you to become your own sleep expert!

Section 3: Techniques to improve your sleep

This is broken down into five short chapters designed to be used over a six-week programme:

1. Week one: First, I will introduce you to the sleep diary and teach you how to measure your own sleep.

2. Week two: Next, we can look at your sleep patterns and the things you do that might be affecting your sleep; this is called 'sleep hygiene'. I will also teach you some ways to relax and wind down before bedtime.

3. Weeks three and four: Then, with all this information in mind, we will take the big step of scheduling a new sleep pattern for you. In doing so we will look at two techniques called 'sleep restriction' and 'stimulus control'. These are challenging but often very effective, so I will be particularly encouraging and motivating over these weeks.

4. Week five: Many people tell me they are

sleepy on the sofa but as soon as they lie down it 'is as if a light is switched on'. They may also talk about a 'racing mind'. If this sounds familiar then there are techniques I can teach you that will help with this.

5. Week six: The relapse prevention toolkit – finally, when your sleep starts to improve, I need to show you how to keep it all going. It is important to plan ahead to stop things slipping backwards. So, this section is all about a longer-term plan to prevent relapse once things are getting better.

Section 4: Recovery stories

In this section, you can see whether Poppy's and Paul's stories sound like yours. I will be honest about some of the difficulties that they had along the way, how they found the different parts of the treatment, and what they did to help their own sleep. Some people like to read this first to know more about the techniques before they start – it can help to know that you are not alone and other people have had the same problems and have got better. You can also see their sleep diaries, which can help you to understand how to use yours.

How to use this book

Before you start I would like to share with you some tips about how best to use self-help. Some of these apply to the use of self-help in general, and not just this book.

Tip 1: Give it your best shot

'I wasn't sure at first, some of the things I was told to do seemed really hard and I waited until after the Christmas holidays before I started the sleep diaries. I am so glad I stuck with it though.'

The programme is laid out over six weeks and week by week we will introduce the techniques that you need to improve your sleep. Having time to read through the material and complete the sleep diaries week by week will really help. So, make sure that this is the best time for you to start therapy. I would suggest avoiding periods where you may have a big commitment at work, or holidays where you might change time zones and bedrooms. Reading the stories of others who have been through the programme may help (see Section 4). Also, you can help to motivate yourself by listing the benefits that you are hoping to gain from the programme (for example, improved concentration or more energy). If you feel your commitment drifting, revisit these benefits or keep them alive by writing them on a Post-it and sticking it to the bathroom mirror or on the fridge. Set aside time, not just before bedtime, to go through the diaries and really allow yourself time to understand and think about the techniques. If you were attending a CBT course, you would need at least one to two hours a week as your homework time. So, allow yourself at least as much time with this book. It may be helpful to plan ahead when would be the best time to do this; maybe it is in the bath in the evening or after your evening meal. Try to find a time that is quiet when you can really concentrate.

Tip 2: Put what you learn into action

'What really helped was starting to write things down, night by night.'

Hopefully, I will be able to explain why I am asking you to change things about your schedule and your patterns. But this is a doing book and not just a reading book! Read it cover to cover first if you wish, but I really want you to start by assessing your sleep and then use this as a manual to change it and improve things.

I will take you through things slowly and step by step, so you don't feel overloaded with too much to try and change too quickly. Remember, this is a week-by-week programme over six to seven weeks to help you sleep better.

Tip 3: Expect to have good and bad days (and nights)

'It was all going really well and then I just lay awake all night after an argument at work; it felt as if all the hard work had been for nothing. But then I went back to my sleep diaries and read through what had fixed things before. The next night I had a plan to get up and out of the bedroom if I couldn't sleep. Just having the plan made me less bothered heading into the bedroom. And it worked; I woke a bit but much less and I wasn't agitated. The night after, I was woken by the alarm!'

Like everyone who goes through this therapy, you will have ups and downs, and some nights will feel easier than others. This is normal, it is surprising just how many good sleepers occasionally have a bad night's sleep. So, don't let one bad night persuade you that things are not working and make you give up. Looking at the pattern over the next few weeks is what matters and over this period of time you should see a gradual improvement. This is one reason why it is helpful to keep a record, as it lets you see this pattern.

Tip 4: Let your GP know that you are going to use the book

'My GP was really supportive, in fact she didn't know much about CBT for insomnia but when I showed her the book she was interested and said she thought it was a good idea. We had talked about sleeping tablets before, but we agreed that we wouldn't change any of my medication until after the programme had finished and then we could talk again. I had wanted to stop some of my tablets in case they were causing the problems with sleep but she explained they weren't, so this was useful. You never know – it might mean she can tell other patients too.'

This treatment has been used safely for many patients but I would still recommend that you let your GP or regular doctor know before you start. It really helps if other things in your life are stable and, in particular, making a plan with your doctor about how to adjust any tablets or medicines that might change your sleep is important. There is a section on sleeping tablets later in the book that might help you to do this. Also, letting your GP know that you are committed to change can help to motivate you.

Tip 5: Involve family and friends if you can

'I know that bad sleep was affecting my relationship. My husband was getting cross when I was up at night and it was disturbing his sleep as well. In fact, he had asked me to go to the doctor. I know it's not fair but when he was sleeping well (and snoring) it just made me even more angry. I told him about the treatment and he was glad I was trying something, in fact he read bits of the book as well.'

Sleep problems can really cause trouble not just for my patients but for their bed partners as well. Sometimes I feel as if it is 'two for the price of one' in the sleep clinic! So, talk through the therapy plan with your family if they are in the house. This can help you to work around your routines but also theirs and it can make a big difference to success rates. Family and friends can keep you going if you are finding things tough. If you show them sections of the book, there is bound to be something about sleep they didn't know and find interesting, so get them on board early. Telling them that you are planning to make changes can help your own motivation as well. We know that someone supporting you to use CBT can make it more effective (it makes it less easy to let things slip).

Getting and using professional support

You may or may not be receiving support to use this book. In NHS England, there are now Improving Access to Psychological Therapies (IAPT) services where people suitable for CBT can be supported to work through psychological problems either by telephone, face-to-face or online. Psychological Wellbeing Practitioners (PWPs) are healthcare practitioners specifically trained to assess and support people in using books such as this one. They can explain anything that you are struggling to understand and help you to put plans into action. If you feel that this form of support would be helpful then, in England, you can usually self-refer to local IAPT services (see: www.nhs.uk/Service-Search and search for 'psychological therapies' or IAPT in your area) or you can ask your GP to refer you.

PWPs also support individuals who experience many different anxiety disorders and also depression. Sleep problems can be linked to these psychological difficulties and your GP or PWP will be able to let you know if this is the case.

Building motivation to change – what do you need from this therapy?

I have worked with lots of patients with bad sleep

and it is really helpful to understand what they want to achieve from therapy before we start. What would you like to achieve over the next six weeks with this book? 'Just to get a good night's sleep' is something I have heard from almost all my patients over the years, but what would this mean to you?

It can be helpful to write this down and think through your own goals and I have left space on pages 16–19 for you to do this. Try to think about things that are specific to you and that you could measure in some way. This can be where the sleep diary comes in because you can start to put some numbers on to your sleep and also measure the problem in a way that you can see. For insomnia, people often want more sleep (eight hours is the number I am asked for most often in the sleep clinic) but they also feel that their sleep quality is poor. Your main priority may be to feel more refreshed when you wake up so that you can cope with the next day. Some people feel that their sleep is not normal any more and just want to be able to sleep as well as their family or friends seem to. When you write down your goals you can come back to them as you are working through therapy to see how you are doing. You can always check back as we go through the book and you can adjust them if you need to. It's a good idea to check them after a month of the therapy, and then again after two and three months.

You can look back at your baseline and where your sleep was when you started. If possible, try to set realistic goals. For example, if you really want to sleep for eight hours but are only sleeping for four hours at present, then would you see progress if you were sleeping six and a half or seven hours a night?

Rating my goals

My goals for feeling better

Goal 1: ....

....

....Today's date __/__/__

I can do this now (circle a number):

0	1	2	3	4	5	6
Not at all		Occasionally		Often		Any time

One month re-rating   (Today's date___/___/___)
(circle a number):

0	1	2	3	4	5	6
Not at all		Occasionally		Often		Any time

Two month re-rating   (Today's date___/___/___)
(circle a number):

0	1	2	3	4	5	6
Not at all		Occasionally		Often		Any time

Three month re-rating   (Today's date___/___/___)
(circle a number):

0	1	2	3	4	5	6
Not at all		Occasionally		Often		Any time

Goal 2: ....

....

....Today's date___/___/___

I can do this now (circle a number):

0	1	2	3	4	5	6
Not at all		Occasionally		Often		Any time

One month re-rating   (Today's date___/___/___)
(circle a number):

0	1	2	3	4	5	6
Not at all		Occasionally		Often		Any time

Two month re-rating   (Today's date___/___/___)
(circle a number):

0	1	2	3	4	5	6
Not at all		Occasionally		Often		Any time

Three month re-rating   (Today's date___/___/___)
(circle a number):

0	1	2	3	4	5	6
Not at all		Occasionally		Often		Any time

Goal 3: ....

....

....Today's date___/___/___

I can do this now (circle a number):

0	1	2	3	4	5	6
Not at all		Occasionally		Often		Any time

One month re-rating   (Today's date___/___/___)
(circle a number):

0	1	2	3	4	5	6
Not at all		Occasionally		Often		Any time

Two month re-rating   (Today's date___/___/___)
(circle a number):

0	1	2	3	4	5	6
Not at all		Occasionally		Often		Any time

Three month re-rating   (Today's date___/___/___)
(circle a number):

0	1	2	3	4	5	6
Not at all		Occasionally		Often		Any time

Section 2

UNDERSTANDING SLEEP: HOW AND WHY WE DO IT, AND WHY DOES IT GO WRONG

We all talk about 'going to sleep' without really thinking much about what that means. The comedian George Carlin famously talked about how bizarre the state of sleep was, temporarily losing command of everything we can do, everything we understand – only for life to start again as normal when the sun comes up. Dreaming of adventures that are impossible in real life but happen each and every night. I think this captures much of what people know and don't know about sleep. If we do think about it at all, it seems a bizarre state of suspended reality. We really don't remember much about the night when we sleep well. For many years it was thought of as a passive state. After all, we still talk about 'going out like a light' or 'switching off' as if a switch just flips us off for the next eight hours, but that is not what happens at all. To help to improve your sleep, it is worth understanding more about its nuts and bolts. In other words, how the brain controls sleep, and how sleep controls the brain.

We now know that distinct areas within the brain control a complex and very active process that changes over the night. If we think of the brain as a series of electrical circuits then there are two separate circuits that control how long we sleep, and why we sleep at night and usually not in the day. I often explain these as the Hours and the Clocks.

The Hours – the sleep homeostat

This is the electrical circuit that drives how many hours we sleep for – we all sleep (honestly). It may feel that you have had little or no sleep because you are reading this, but sleep is a necessity for all of us. We can sleep badly but we all sleep at some stage and there is a pressure to sleep that builds up with every hour we have been awake. So, the longer we are awake, the sleepier we become. When we do sleep, that pressure to sleep decreases to then build up again over the hours once we are awake again. This is called the homeostat. We can think of this a bit like the thermostat for the heating in your house. The thermostat keeps the system balanced and makes the house warmer when the weather is cold and turns itself off when it is too hot.

Lots of other systems in the body are regulated in the same way. So with hunger, the longer you wait between meals, the hungrier you become. However, you are not hungry immediately after eating or much less hungry if you snack before dinner. For most of us, the drive for sleep becomes strong enough after about sixteen hours awake that we then sleep for seven to eight hours. This also means that if you have a nap during the day, then you will not be quite as sleepy at your normal bedtime.

The Clocks – the circadian rhythm

We live on a planet that rotates around the sun every twenty-four hours, and every bit of our biology is designed around this day and night cycle. Our bodies have many 'circadian' rhythms (circadian means 'about a day'), although we often neglect them in our modern 24/7 culture. We know that supermarkets, gyms and coffee shops can all be open twenty-four hours a day and the seductive charms of the internet can make it seem like permanent daytime.

The Biological Clock

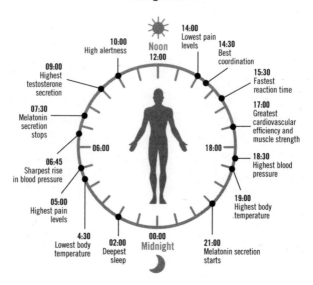

One of the most important circadian rhythms is the sleep-wake cycle. Humans are designed for daytime activity and night-time sleep. In addition, there is a natural peak in sleepiness mid-afternoon; this is why in some hot countries, a siesta takes place then.

We can see from the diagram of the biological clock above that all of our body systems – reaction speed, body temperature or when we feel most sleepy – vary over the twenty-four hours. A tiny area deep within the brain (called the suprachiasmatic nucleus or SCN), sends signals to the brain and the rest of the body and controls the body clock and the sleep-wake cycle. It acts a little bit like the conductor of an orchestra – keeping everything to time. The single most important timekeeper for the SCN is **light.** Specialised cells in the retina at the back of the eye measure the light intensity or exactly how bright it is and send signals to the SCN. We feel much more sleepy in the dark and more alert in bright light. So, our sleep-wake cycle is hardwired to light and, therefore, the time of day.

Clearly there are other things that can disrupt and override these signals. For example, we can all work shifts or get up to look after our children at night if we need to. However, the artificial light in our offices and houses usually has a much lower intensity than natural light. This will make you feel sluggish, more fatigued and less alert working indoors compared to being outdoors. People with insomnia often focus on the night hours but, as night follows day, we can see that daytime light and activity levels will have a big effect on sleep as well.

Understanding both the homeostat (the Hours) and the circadian rhythm (the Clock) helps us to understand why we are most likely to fall asleep:

- When we are really sleepy and have been awake for some time.

- At night and in the dark and at roughly the same time each day.

When sleep goes wrong a number of things tend to happen. We need sleep to feel well and so we often feel fatigued and grumpy when we sleep badly. People notice that their attention and concentration are not as good during the day. However, this can lead to us changing what we do in and out of the bedroom to try and get a better night. Although this is understandable, some of the things we do might actually make sleep worse and this can lead to a vicious circle with a downward spiral. People can become increasingly anxious about the process of falling asleep itself. We all tend to feel more awake and alert when we are anxious, exactly the opposite of what we need at bedtime. So the feelings of tension and frustration if you can't sleep can start to affect behaviour in the bedroom and what you are thinking when you are lying in bed.

Meet Poppy and Paul

People who are struggling to sleep often want to know that they are not alone (particularly at four in the morning!) and it can be useful to read about other people with the same problems. It is particularly useful if they have used self-help CBT for insomnia successfully, so I want to introduce you to Poppy and Paul. They were both having poor sleep.

Poppy's story

Poppy was thirty-two and had just returned to work after having her first son Sam. She was married to Mike, worked as a teaching assistant in a primary school and she loved it. Life felt busy now Sam was around. He went to the local nursery, with Mum helping out with some of the drop-offs. She had always been a light sleeper but, after Sam was born, the first few months made her really tired. She couldn't wait for him to sleep a few hours without waking her, but he seemed to take months longer to sleep through compared to her friends' children.

But now, thank goodness, he did drop off to sleep easily and so she just couldn't understand why she wasn't sleeping like she did before he was born. At first, it was just occasional nights when she got into bed feeling awake, tired but wired. And it seemed to take so long; her husband fell asleep as soon as his head hit the pillow. She had never noticed his breathing before and his snoring. It just seemed to be rubbing in the fact she was awake.

Then it was most nights and even when she did fall asleep, she would wake again. Even if Sam was asleep and her husband was snoring. Everything seemed uncomfortable and she was too hot or too cold. Sometimes she got up and once she tried doing all the ironing – she thought at least if she was awake she might as well be productive. In fact, the only time she felt like sleeping was when the alarm finally went off at 6.30. She started to feel more and more tired. Sometimes she would fall asleep watching TV and then when she did get into bed it was even harder to get to sleep.

She knew that she was feeling more irritable and short-tempered with Sam and Mike and the worse the night was, the worse she felt the next day. Sometimes counting down the hours just felt like torture. She tried herbal remedies from the pharmacist, different pillows and even the spare room but none of it worked.

When she went to her GP she was first given a short leaflet on stopping coffee and other advice that didn't really seem to apply to her. When she went back she felt desperate for a better solution, just one good night. The GP said that she could try some sleeping tablets but they didn't tend to fix the problem long-term. Now she had been sleeping badly for over six months. He did say that there was a type of CBT that helped and a self-help book could take her through this. He explained it was different to the things that she might have read before because it would let her measure her sleep and then help work out a plan for in the bedroom.

She was sceptical at first because she just wanted a quick fix, she felt she had waited a long time and she worried about bad sleep stopping her doing her job properly. But, after she started reading the book, she looked up some of the other information on the NHS websites and lots of people said it worked. She started to understand how some of the things she had been doing to try and get a better night might actually have been making things worse and not better. You can find out how she started to record her sleep problem and how the therapy went in Section 4.

Paul's story

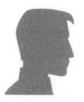

Paul was forty-two and worked as a sales rep in a local office. He had never had a problem with sleep before and then he caught the flu. It was the same bug that his wife and both of the children had but he had two weeks with chills and feeling awful. He stopped going to the gym because he felt really achy. He was back to work after three weeks, but for the first few nights after he got back he felt restless and much more wide awake than usual. His wife had suggested going to bed early, she thought he might still be run-down after the flu.

He lay in bed next to her an hour earlier than his usual bedtime but he couldn't sleep. It felt odd – she normally teased him for falling asleep on the sofa too late. On the fourth night he just couldn't fall asleep, the harder he tried and the longer he lay there, the more cross he got. He went downstairs and immediately fell asleep on the sofa watching an old film. The next night he tried again to get into bed when his wife went up but he still couldn't fall asleep straight away. This time he got straight back up and put the TV on; the problem was the sofa was pretty uncomfortable so he fell asleep but woke up a bit cross with a sore neck. Then when he went back into the bedroom he lay awake again, this time it was three in the morning. He started to think about the next day at work, it was a big regional meeting. He knew that he got a headache when he slept badly and he really wanted to do well at the meeting. Eventually he went downstairs and had a large brandy and that seemed to work.

Next day's meeting went badly. He still had a headache and quite suddenly he seemed to have a sleep problem. He began to try and catch up on his sleep at the weekends by lying in. During the week he often didn't go up to bed until after the second or even third film, but lay dozing on the sofa. It was starting to put a strain on his relationship with his wife, and his family now had to tiptoe around the house in the mornings.

Now everywhere he seemed to look, people were sleeping well or telling him how tired he looked. His wife told him to go to the doctor. He didn't really want to for something as trivial as a bad night but, after a year, he finally went. He was getting so tired he thought he wouldn't be safe driving.

The GP went through things. She thought his mood was a bit low but his main problem was the insomnia. She also told him that he was drinking too much. She said she couldn't give him sleeping tablets if he was drinking and it might make him feel sleepy behind the wheel. She did say he might still be able to sort things out himself if he cut down on his alcohol, but he felt a bit cross and thought there must still be some lingering infection after the flu or that there was a medical problem. The GP did do some blood tests and said they were all fine and she thought he should try working with a counsellor who could help him with his sleep. She sent him to see someone called Rekke, a Psychological Wellbeing Practitioner (PWP). She seemed very straightforward and said that she had worked with lots of people who had bad insomnia. She explained that although he wasn't deliberately trying to disrupt his sleep, some of the things he was doing to try to cope were actually making things worse. She started to talk about a time when his sleeping was fine and asked him how he went to bed and fell asleep back then. He didn't know and she said that was part of the point. Sleep was an automatic process and thinking about it sometimes meant you were putting a lot of effort into it, which made it hard work. She gave him other examples of things he did best automatically like controlling his breathing. When she started talking about his breathing, it made him start to take deep breaths which felt odd and a bit uncomfortable, so what she was saying made sense. She gave him a sleep diary to fill in and said this would help her look at some of his sleep routines in a bit more detail so she could help him. You can find out how he started to tackle his bad nights and late films on page 139.

What actually happens when you sleep?

In the sleep clinic, we can record sleep and look at the electrical activity in the brain (the EEG). We can see that there are two main stages of sleep; dream sleep (also known as REM sleep) and non-dream sleep (NREM or deep sleep, sometimes called slow-wave sleep). Most of our dream sleep comes in the second half of the night. Recording sleep in the hospital tells us some really interesting things about sleep. We tend to go between non-dream and dream sleep in approximately ninety-minute cycles. The diagram below shows this in a little more detail.

Hypnogram of Normal Sleep

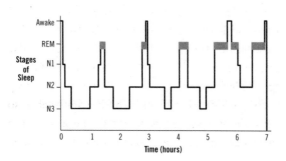

It may be a surprise to know that everybody wakes up during the night. Two to four times at least, even in young and healthy people, and up to six to eight times for people over the age of sixty. We all tend to wake more in the second half of the night and it is much easier to wake someone from dream sleep. So now we know that nobody 'sleeps through' the night, even if you do not have insomnia. In fact, everybody wakes during the night. Most people do not remember these wakenings or they are very short and they go straight back to sleep.

Why do we sleep?

> 'Sleep is the cement that sticks our days together.'
>
> – Rob Auton, *Take Hair* (2017)

Sleep is vital for our mood, memory and metabolism. All three of these things rely on normal quantities of sleep and they all suffer if we sleep badly for any reason. Much of our understanding of what sleep does comes from research that deprives people of sleep and then studies the effects of this on physical and mental health. We have known for some time that sleep is necessary for every aspect of daytime life and we simply can't do without it. Let's look at the results of this research in a bit more detail.

Our mood and mental health depend on sleep, and this relationship works in both directions. The very first signs of depression or anxiety can be a broken and fragmented night. However, insomnia itself increases the risk of depression. People who have suffered from depression and then recovered are more likely to relapse if they have insomnia. One study that followed young adults with persistent insomnia showed that these people were seven times more likely to develop depression when compared to a similar group who slept well.

One of the most striking effects of loss of sleep is poor attention, but poor memory is also an issue. This is not just because we get too sleepy during the day to concentrate properly. Sleep plays a really important role in consolidating all of our new memories, so the things that we learn during the day are replayed at night to help us store them within our memory. This might be one reason that you need to go through this book a few times!

How much sleep do you need?

Just as we know that some people are short and some are tall, we all need different amounts of sleep. It is true to say that most adults over the age of twenty-five need about seven to eight hours of sleep. Research shows that if people are left to fall asleep and wake without an alarm, then this is the average amount of sleep that they report. Equally, a small number of people really seem wide awake and refreshed after only five or six hours' sleep. In contrast, some people only feel refreshed with nine or even ten hours' sleep. However, very few people are truly refreshed after only four hours. There are a few myths associated with famous short sleepers such as Margaret Thatcher and Napoleon but, in fact, they both took daytime power naps to catch up.

In the same way, the body clock (circadian rhythm) varies across the population. Most adults will be most likely to fall asleep at about 11 p.m. and wake around 7 a.m. However, 5–10 per cent of us are night owls who go to sleep well after midnight but wake up later in the morning. In contrast, about 10 per cent of us are morning larks feeling sleepy long before midnight but comfortable waking up between 5 or 6 a.m. It is worth thinking about when you were most likely to fall asleep before you had trouble sleeping. Were you a lark or an owl or somewhere in the middle?

Sleep is also flexible, so when normal sleepers are studied over time they sleep different amounts of time over the week. Again, this is normal and so you shouldn't expect to have exactly the same amount of sleep each night. Most of us are aware that we sleep a little longer at the weekends or on holidays. We also sleep more if we are ill, particularly if we have a temperature. This is part of recovery as key parts of the immune system are active during sleep.

There are interesting changes to sleep that occur over the course of our lives. Very young children typically sleep many more hours than adults, although not always at the times that suit their parents! Your total sleep time decreases throughout childhood, increases a little to an average of eight to ten hours in teenagers (coinciding with the final growth spurt at the end of puberty – we produce more growth hormone at night). As we age, we sleep less, and the average amount of time that older adults spend asleep is six to six and a half hours. It is also normal for older adults to sleep less deeply than younger adults, with less deep sleep and increased night wakenings. We are generally easier to wake later in life, so sleep is more easily broken.

There is also a change in the pattern of sleep as we get older. We have a natural tendency to fall asleep earlier with each decade that passes (so we tend to become morning larks rather than night owls). Teenagers are set to fall asleep later than their parents and most are night owls falling asleep after midnight, this is with or without their phones and laptops. Older adults may be much more comfortable falling asleep closer to 10 p.m. and rising between 5 and 6 a.m.

Are there good and bad sleepers?

Many people in the clinic describe themselves as bad sleepers, others will say they are good sleepers. Equally, quite a few of my patients have not really thought about their sleep at all – usually the good sleepers! As I have said, most of us do not think about sleep until it goes wrong. At best it is an automatic act. The truth is that most people have both good and bad nights, so even good sleepers will recognise the occasional bad night. However, those with insomnia tend to report most nights as bad – typically three or more a week.

What is insomnia?

People with insomnia have difficulty falling asleep or difficulty staying asleep ... or more often both! Some people also feel that their sleep is non-restorative, so they do manage to get to sleep but feel their sleep is not 'a proper sleep' and they do not feel refreshed on waking.

This needs to be three or more nights a week, in other words to be a regular part of life, to be classed as insomnia. Most people with insomnia will take more than thirty minutes to fall asleep and then will be awake in the night for more than thirty minutes. The box below summarises how I diagnose insomnia when I see people in the sleep clinic. You can see that insomnia must have been a problem for at least three months and must also cause problems during the day. This is important because people tend to ask for help with insomnia because of the effect it has on the next day. They may complain of poor concentration, irritability or feel less productive in day-to-day life.

Insomnia

- Difficulty falling asleep and/or difficulty staying asleep.
- The poor sleep is causing a problem during the day – poor concentration, fatigue or distress.
- It happens at least three or more nights a week.
- It has been happening for at least three months.
- It is not due to another physical cause of bad sleep.

What causes insomnia to become a long-term problem?

An occasional bad night is normal for all of us, but why do some people develop persistent insomnia?

We know that some people are predisposed to develop insomnia, so this might be a genetic tendency. Insomnia can run in families, and some people recognise they are light sleepers just as their parents are. However, there is often some kind of trigger. This could be a physical illness, something as simple as a different sleeping environment, anxiety or some daytime stresses, for example an approaching exam or holiday with a time-zone change. When I introduced you to one of our cases, Poppy, it was her son being born and then returning to work that changed routines around and which was the start of the problem. She was always a light sleeper but things became much worse over a few months.

However, for insomnia to be a long-term problem, the key seems to be perpetuating factors (these are things we do that tend to keep the problem going). For example, when the bed is no longer a relaxing place but starts to cause stress, going to bed then starts to cause anxiety. Becoming anxious about sleep can in itself worsen sleep as heart rate, adrenaline levels and blood pressure all increase, and these are things that make us feel awake. People with insomnia can often then change their sleep routines to try and catch up on sleep or improve things, but paradoxically this can make things worse and not better. For example, people might go to bed earlier to try and catch up on sleep but this leads to longer lying in bed awake and increases stress and frustration. Patterns of thinking about sleep then change over time – you can see this when you look at the diagram below. Sleep really works best when we don't think about it at all.

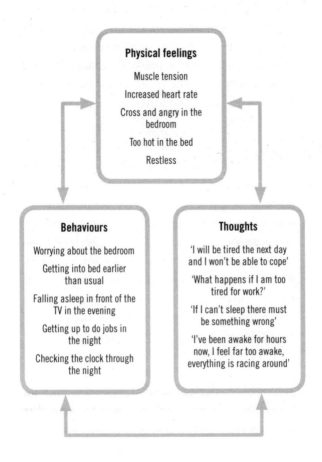

Physical feelings

Muscle tension

Increased heart rate

Cross and angry in the bedroom

Too hot in the bed

Restless

Behaviours

Worrying about the bedroom

Getting into bed earlier than usual

Falling asleep in front of the TV in the evening

Getting up to do jobs in the night

Checking the clock through the night

Thoughts

'I will be tired the next day and I won't be able to cope'

'What happens if I am too tired for work?'

'If I can't sleep there must be something wrong'

'I've been awake for hours now, I feel far too awake, everything is racing around'

What is the link between insomnia and other illnesses?

Insomnia can be linked to mental health problems but also to other illness. Arthritis might cause pain at night, asthma could cause breathlessness, as a couple of examples. If there is chronic poor sleep with these problems then this is called comorbid insomnia. This simply means insomnia alongside another illness.

It is important also to say that insomnia does not have to be caused by any of these problems. Many people are frustrated by doctors or other health professionals assuming that all of their sleep problems are caused by depression or a physical health problem such as arthritis, and they can feel that the insomnia is not being taking seriously as a problem in its own right. Luckily, there is good evidence that the techniques I will teach you work both for insomnia and comorbid insomnia.

Should I take medication for insomnia?

Traditionally, doctors have prescribed medication for insomnia. However, we now know that sleeping tablets should really only be used for short-term insomnia of more than three months. Usually your doctor will only want to prescribe these tablets for two weeks, and no longer, because they can cause side effects. They do seem to help when there has been a specific trigger to poor sleep. If the tablets are used for longer than this, the initial benefits of them often wear off. Some people do not find them helpful and they can cause a grogginess and a 'hangover effect' in the morning. Many people are now aware that these drugs can be addictive. Certain other medications, in particular antidepressants, are also used 'off licence' to treat insomnia, but there are very few good research studies to say that these drugs will work well in the long term. The treatment with the best evidence for success is CBTi, in other words the techniques that this book will teach you. This is now the recommended treatment within the NHS (www.nhs.uk/conditions/Insomnia).

Sleeping pills

The first and most important point to make is always to discuss any tablets that you take with your doctor and that will usually be your GP. Your doctor knows your background medical details and the reasons for the tablets you are prescribed. This is the best person to give advice about all of your pills, including any that you may take to try and help you sleep.

However, we can make some general points about sleeping tablets. Many patients come to me having tried sleeping pills. Some are still on them when they come to the sleep clinic and some want to use the CBT programme to come off sleeping tablets. You may have a number of questions about your tablets and this programme. First of all, I have written down a brief description of the tablets that your GP can prescribe for you to try and help you to sleep. Some of these tablets are also used for other conditions such as depression or to help with pain. We need to know about something called the 'half-life' of a drug. This is the time your body takes to remove half of the drug from the bloodstream. For sleeping tablets, it helps to know 1) how quickly they work to get into your system when you first take them and 2) how long it takes for your body to remove them.

Table for sleeping tablets

Name	Dose range (mg)	Half-life (hours)	Common side effects
Zopiclone	3.75–15	4–6	Morning hangover
Temazepam	5–20	6–8	Morning hangover
Zolpidem	5–20	2–4	Headache, sleepwalking
Clonazepam	0.5–1	10–17	Daytime sleepiness, worse snoring
Melatonin	2	0.5–2	Headache, low mood
Amitriptyline	10–50	17	Dry mouth, morning hangover
Mirtazepine	15–45	20–40	Weight gain, worsen restless legs
Trazodone	50–200	10–12	Weight gain

Understanding a bit about how sleeping tablets work may well help you to make decisions about the tablets. There is surprisingly little evidence that sleeping tablets are helpful for chronic insomnia; this is insomnia that has lasted over three months. This statement is based on a large number of research papers where the evidence has been carefully studied. Most of the research has shown that sleeping tablets taken for a few days and up to three to four weeks can help people to fall asleep quicker and sometimes to stay asleep a bit longer. However, they also show that the tablets can cause people to feel a little groggy and hungover in the morning, so some people can feel that insomnia has made them feel fatigued when in fact the lingering effects of the sleeping tablet can be part of the problem.

Sometimes the tablets work for a short time but people then develop a tolerance to them. In other words, the initial benefit seems to fade quite quickly and they need to take a higher dose to get the same benefit. This can lead to the worst of all worlds with the drug seeming to stop working to help you fall asleep, but then to cause insomnia that is even worse when trying to stop it. If you are prescribed the drugs, the best way to try and avoid tolerance is to use the tablets for short periods, and this is why doctors will now often prescribe them for two weeks at a time but not for any longer.

Can I use the CBT to help me come off sleeping tablets?

The short answer is yes you can but again this has to be done with a discussion first with your GP or regular doctor to make sure that they agree and think that this is safe. We find that people do best making a clear timetable and working out what would suit them best. This will be different for different people. After all, you may well have friends who stopped smoking. Some will have cut down gradually and others stopped straight away but used a support group or medication. Similarly, there are different ways to stop sleeping tablets and you need to find the best way for you. If you are only taking the tablets occasionally and not every day, one plan would be to stop when you start the sleep restriction part of the programme (within Section 3).

The alternative is to keep your tablets exactly as they are and work through the programme first. The advantage here would be that you don't have to worry about the effects of coming off the tablets and can really concentrate on the sleep therapy itself. Lots of the people who see me in clinic are really bothered about the idea of stopping the tablets and having withdrawal symptoms. They worry that things will get even worse. I often suggest putting that to one side entirely, simply starting the sleep diary and getting on with the programme.

Possibly the most important thing is to make a plan and try to stick to it. Make the plan that suits both you and your doctor. The one thing that can disrupt the CBTi programme is changing the tablets or the dose of your tablets half way through therapy. So, decide which plan you will be able to stick with and talk to your GP. The key thing is that most people want an alternative to sleeping tablets because they are unhappy with them in some way. So, if that applies to you, make a plan and try this programme. We know that it has worked for many others.

Could it be another sleep problem?

This is a really important question. Insomnia is not the only problem people can have with their sleep. The techniques I am going to teach you work really well for people with insomnia but they may not help with other sleep problems. So, this section aims to give you some information about the other sleep disorders. Now I am not saying that you should be diagnosing your own illness – doctors and other health professionals are trained to go through your symptoms to work out which disease you have (the diagnosis). They often go through a number of questions and may arrange tests to work out the difference between different diseases. This process usually starts with a meeting with your GP.

Certain questions help your GP work out which problem you have. Sometimes they may refer you to see a hospital-based sleep specialist like myself. Some of these questions are listed below and can give you some more information about different types of sleep problems and help you find the right professional help. You may have more than one sleep disorder.

Q1. When you try to relax in the evening or sleep at night, do you ever have unpleasant, restless feelings in your legs that can be relieved by walking or movement?

Restless legs syndrome (RLS) and periodic limb movements of sleep

This is a common condition, with at least 5 per cent of the population recognising an odd, fidgety irritable feeling in their legs that makes them want to get up, stretch, move or kick. This does not always disturb sleep but some people have more severe restless legs that quite literally do not let them rest. This is a secondary cause of insomnia. In my clinic at least 10 per cent of all the patients sent to me with insomnia either have restless legs as their main problem or have restless legs on some nights that disturb sleep. Restless legs tend to be worse late evening or in the first half of the night.

If you think restless legs are disturbing your sleep, it is worth talking to your doctor about these symptoms. A bed partner may be able to tell you that your legs twitch or jerk even when you have drifted off (it may really annoy them!).

Not everyone with restless legs needs medical treatment and some people know that their RLS only occurs occasionally, but some simple lifestyle measures that tend to help include avoiding caffeine, nicotine (smoking or vaping) and alcohol late into the evening. All of these things tend to make RLS worse. Some people who make the really positive step of stopping smoking will often notice that their legs feel less irritable and sleep is better.

There is a link between RLS and low iron levels and so sometimes your GP may ask for a blood test to measure your iron levels. It is also worth looking at any medications you may be prescribed for other reasons. Certain tablets can make RLS worse and this includes some of the antidepressant drugs, melatonin and some anti-sickness tablets, so asking your GP about this can be helpful. RLS-UK is a helpful medical charity with some useful patient information. For persistent and severe restless legs, certain medications can be very effective but your GP will need to discuss with you whether these will be suitable. The NHS Choices website can also provide some helpful information.

Q2. When you do get to sleep, do you snore loudly? Do you feel very sleepy during the day?

Obstructive sleep apnoea (OSA)

Other people's snoring can disturb your sleep and some people with insomnia can be particularly frustrated by a bed partner's loud snores. However, you might not have thought about your own snoring or breathing as being a part of your bad night's sleep.

We know at least 20 per cent of the population snore and for many of them it is simply a nuisance to others. However, for some, loud snoring can be associated with pauses in the breathing (apnoeas) when no air passes in or out for a few seconds. This disturbs sleep much more as it tends to cause brief wakenings and a very broken night. People can be entirely unaware of these wakenings and simply feel horribly unrefreshed by their sleep ('as if I haven't been to bed' can be what patients tell me). Clues can be a sore dry throat in the morning and a dull headache. Some people are more aware that they wake at night, occasionally with a feeling of choking or increased need to pass urine.

The key difference between insomnia and a broken night caused by OSA is usually daytime sleepiness. Those with moderate or severe OSA will typically struggle to get though the day without actually napping or dozing. Many people have OSA that is undiagnosed. In fact at least 10 per cent of men and 5 per cent of women over the age of forty have some level of OSA. This makes it one of the commonest sleep problems. The good news is that there is an effective treatment to stop the snoring and pauses in breathing (a device you can wear called CPAP). This makes your sleep a lot better.

The biggest risk factor for snoring is neck circumference (your collar size) and your weight or Body Mass Index (BMI; you can calculate this using the simple NHS calculator available on the internet). Unfortunately, obesity has risen in the population from 15 per cent in the 1990s to 25 per cent of the general population in 2015. It is worth asking your bedpartner (if you have one) about any snoring or pauses in your breathing. There are some simple screening tools available, and some more information about obstructive sleep apnoea can be found in the Resources section at the end of this book.

Q3. Do you sleep well but it seems to be at the wrong time?

Circadian rhythm disorders

We talked about the body clock that regulates when we fall asleep. Some people have circadian rhythm disorders and simply feel very wide awake late at night, but can fall asleep well if they are allowed to go to bed when they want – for example at 3 a.m. However, they then really struggle to wake for school or get to work at 8 a.m! This is different to insomnia. A condition called Delayed Sleep Phase Syndrome leads to people being extreme night owls, most comfortable falling asleep between 3 and 4 a.m., but then sleeping long and deep into normal waking time. Advanced Sleep Phase Syndrome is a similar problem with the body clock but with the opposite effect. People simply can't stay awake late at all and may go to bed very early, then wake well before 5 a.m. and be unable to return to sleep.

Q4. Do you sleepwalk or have vivid unpleasant dreams that wake you?

Parasomnias

These are any unwanted behaviours or activities coming from sleep. This might include sleepwalking, sleeptalking, acting out dreams, grinding your teeth loudly or vivid nightmares that are upsetting. Sometimes these are things that happen that your bed partner or other family members tell you about, but you might not remember them properly or the memory of them is confused.

Insomnia can make these problems worse but if this is your main problem, you need to talk to your GP or health professional as there are also other special investigations and treatments that might be needed. There are other psychological therapies that can help with nightmares.

Q5. Do you frequently fall irresistibly asleep during the day with little or no warning?

Narcolepsy

This is a rare condition that typically comes on during the teenage years or early twenties, but it can take a little time to diagnose. Although many people with narcolepsy have a broken night and wake very frequently, they also have a number of other problems including very significant daytime sleepiness and really vivid dreams. Most individuals with narcolepsy will sleep but it can be at times when most of us would be awake (for instance, in an important work meeting, while eating or even talking to people). Their dreams are typically very vivid and memorable most nights, and some people can describe a problem called sleep paralysis. This is waking from a dream but for a minute or so being unable to move at all. It often comes with a feeling of pressure on the chest or a dream-like presence of a figure in the room. People can find sleep paralysis really unpleasant but it is a benign problem and I can reassure you that you will always wake up and be able to move again. Very occasional sleep paralysis can occur in up to 20 per cent of the population but if you have frequent sleep paralysis and very vivid dreams with daytime sleepiness, then you should talk to your GP.

TECHNIQUES TO IMPROVE YOUR SLEEP

Well done for making it this far! Hopefully there has been some helpful information about sleep and insomnia, and also a little about treatment that can help. Now I want to teach you how to start to look at your own sleep and use some specific therapy to help your insomnia. This will help you work towards the goals that you identified in Section 1. Remember that you can make notes in the book, fold down or mark bits that particularly apply to you, and go back at any stage to remind yourself about the previous information we have covered.

The therapy itself is broken down into short sections and tends to work best if you follow the plan week by week over the next six weeks. We are first going to assess your particular insomnia problem. To do this you will learn about measuring your sleep using a sleep diary. Then you have some work to do! These techniques are most effective when they are used together over the six-week programme rather than picking and choosing different things to use independently.

'But I've tried everything' is something I hear every week in the sleep clinic. What most people have not done is really look hard at their own sleep patterns and, over a period of weeks, start to reset their schedule back to a pattern of better sleep. The research into insomnia also shows us that these techniques work whether you have had insomnia for weeks or months or years.

Week 1 – Assessing and measuring your sleep

In this section, I want to introduce a really important tool that we use in the sleep clinic, the sleep diary. This is something I am going to ask you to fill in every day for the next seven days. It is an important starting point for treatment and therapy. I've prepared a blank diary very similar to the ones we use in our sleep clinic to start to put your insomnia into numbers (in the Resources section, pages 145–65).

ACTIVITIES

A	–	each alcoholic drink
C	–	each caffeinated drink, including coffee, tea, chocolate, cola
P	–	every time you take a sleeping pill
M	–	meals
S	–	snacks
X	–	exercise
T	–	use of toilet during sleep-time
N	–	noise that disturbs your sleep
W	–	time of wake-up alarm (if any)

SLEEP TIME (including naps)

↓	–	mark with a 'down' arrow each time you got into bed
↑	–	mark with an 'up' arrow each time you got out of bed
|	–	mark with a line the time you began and the time you ended your sleep; then join the line to indicate sleep periods
|	–	mark with a line the time you began and the time you ended any naps, either in the chair or in bed; then join up lines with a broken line to indicate nap periods

Week 1

	p.m.						midnight / a.m.												noon / p.m.					
	6	7	8	9	10	11	12	1	2	3	4	5	6	7	8	9	10	11	12	1	2	3	4	5	6
Activities																									
Sleep Time																									

LIGHTS OUT_____ a.m. / p.m.   TOTAL SLEEP TIME_____ hrs

	6	7	8	9	10	11	12	1	2	3	4	5	6	7	8	9	10	11	12	1	2	3	4	5	6
Activities																									
Sleep Time																									

LIGHTS OUT_____ a.m. / p.m.   TOTAL SLEEP TIME_____ hrs

	6	7	8	9	10	11	12	1	2	3	4	5	6	7	8	9	10	11	12	1	2	3	4	5	6
Activities																									
Sleep Time																									

LIGHTS OUT_____ a.m. / p.m.   TOTAL SLEEP TIME_____ hrs

	p.m.						midnight / a.m.												noon / p.m.						
	6	7	8	9	10	11	12	1	2	3	4	5	6	7	8	9	10	11	12	1	2	3	4	5	6
Activities																									
Sleep Time																									

LIGHTS OUT_____a.m. / p.m.   TOTAL SLEEP TIME_____ hrs

	p.m.						midnight / a.m.												noon / p.m.						
	6	7	8	9	10	11	12	1	2	3	4	5	6	7	8	9	10	11	12	1	2	3	4	5	6
Activities																									
Sleep Time																									

LIGHTS OUT_____a.m. / p.m.   TOTAL SLEEP TIME_____ hrs

	p.m.						midnight / a.m.												noon / p.m.						
	6	7	8	9	10	11	12	1	2	3	4	5	6	7	8	9	10	11	12	1	2	3	4	5	6
Activities																									
Sleep Time																									

LIGHTS OUT_____a.m. / p.m.   TOTAL SLEEP TIME_____ hrs

	p.m.						midnight / a.m.												noon / p.m.						
	6	7	8	9	10	11	12	1	2	3	4	5	6	7	8	9	10	11	12	1	2	3	4	5	6
Activities																									
Sleep Time																									

LIGHTS OUT_____a.m. / p.m.   TOTAL SLEEP TIME_____ hrs

So you will see that I want you to fill in the diary once a day and ideally, soon after you have woken up in the morning. Write down both when you went to bed and turned the lights out to go to sleep, and then your best guess as to how long it took you to fall asleep. Try to write this down to the nearest five to ten minutes if possible. If you did wake in the middle of the night, jot down how long for and whether you got out of bed (using the arrows). Write down when you woke up and when you got out of bed and what you did using arrows. Extra information includes whether you did any exercise during the day (mark an X), had any drinks with alcohol in them (put an A) and whether you took any sleeping pills (a P). For alcohol, one 'A' would be a single unit (half a pint of beer or a glass of wine). You can put extra notes in if it was an unusual day in some way, for example you were ill. It may be helpful at this point to see how Poppy first filled in her sleep diary as an example to show you how it works (pages 80–81).

I know this may seem like quite a bit of work, so why am I asking you to do it? Well, I usually find that people learn a lot about their own sleep problem from keeping the diary in the first place. Your sleep pattern may be exactly what you expect, but sometimes the pattern looks different or changes more than you realised night to night. Also, I am making this treatment as personalised as possible to your particular sleep problem, exactly as I do in the sleep clinic. So, this is the best way of looking at your problem to then design the best therapy to improve your sleep. This is the information you will use to plan your new schedule and find the best way to beat your insomnia.

I will want you to keep the diary for the next six weeks as you work through the treatment programme. I will be honest and say that this may seem a challenge at times. It is easy to forget to complete the diary during a busy day, but many years of sleep research have shown just how important this part of the programme is. Many patients tell me how much they would give for more sleep. Think of your sleep diary as the price of a better night! The sleep diary is also the way that you will be able to see clearly whether the treatment is working and improving your sleep.

Tips for filling in the sleep diary

1. **Do** fill it in every day, set aside at least few minutes, ideally within the first hour of waking up. Put in as much detail as you remember.

2. **Don't** do this in the middle of the night or clock watch to get the times exact!

3. **Do** write on the diaries that I have given you in the book. There are enough for the whole programme, but if you prefer to keep a notebook or keep rough notes and then put them into the diary, that is fine too. Pen and paper tends to be best rather than apps on your phone as apps don't always have all of the information we need.

4. **Don't** worry about what you put in the diaries themselves; everyone will have different days and different nights and there are no right or wrong things to write down. Your sleep problem is personal to you, so I just need you to tell me about your patterns at the moment.

When you have your sleep diary in front of you and you have written down what has happened over the seven days and nights, it is worth just thinking back to the goals I asked you to write down. Are you ready to change? Now we have put your sleep into numbers, is it what you expected? For example, are all of your nights the same and are they as bad as you thought? Just writing down your patterns is a really important part of therapy, and this first week of keeping the diary is going to help you to start to analyse your sleep and wake patterns in more detail.

Many patients do feel that they have already worked hard at sleep and have had previous disappointments, maybe with tablets or things that seemed to work for other people. So, it is worth thinking about your motivation levels at the moment. There will be some tough changes ahead and it is normal for the path to be bumpy at times, with progress but also occasional relapses. Some people find it helpful to read about the stories of the others we have helped before they start the therapy. Some simply want to get going with their diary in front of them.

Summary of week 1 – the sleep diary

This shows you how to put some numbers on to the problem and with the sleep diary, you can now start to look at your sleep patterns. It will be important to continue to keep the sleep diary over the next five weeks. To move on, it is going to be really helpful to have your diary in front of you with at least seven days and nights filled in.

Week 2 – Sleep hygiene and relaxation

Sleep hygiene

This term is used when we think about your lifestyle and habits during the day that might affect your sleep, your routine before bed and what you do in the bedroom itself. It is a slightly odd term but it is nothing to do with brushing your teeth, having a bath or really clean sheets!

You may have wondered why the diary asks about lots of things that you do in the day when the problem is at night? Some people have already thought hard about the things they might be doing to worsen sleep. In fact, many of my patients with insomnia have already done a lot of research before they meet me. However, it is still worth just going through some of the things you do during the day that might be affecting you at night. You can have a healthy lifestyle and still have insomnia, but some things you do might affect your sleep more than you realise. So, take the time to read through the section below. Your diary may show patterns in your lifestyle that could be making your sleep worse. Over this week, I am going to ask you to make some changes both to your days and what you do in and around the bedroom.

What you do during the day
Caffeine

Most people know that caffeine is a stimulant and makes you feel more awake. That is exactly why we often like it first thing in the morning. The hundreds of coffee shops all over the country show how much we all like both its taste and the mental buzz it provides. You may well have friends who are irritatingly good sleepers but still drink lots of coffee and tea. However, if you have insomnia (remember we talked about having a predisposition or natural tendency to poor or light sleep) then caffeine can and often does keep you awake.

It is worth thinking about the number of cups of tea and coffee you drink but also some of the things that might have hidden caffeine – this includes painkillers, a whole variety of soft drinks, or dark chocolate. The table below shows the amount of caffeine contained in some common drinks and foods (data from http://cspinet.org/eating-healthy/ingredients-of-concern/caffeine-chart).

Substance	Amount of caffeine (mg)
Single shot of expresso (high street coffee)	100mg (range 80–175mg)
Large mug of brewed coffee	95mg
Tea (stewed for 3 minutes)	22–74mg
Coca-Cola	34–70mg
Energy drink (for example, Red Bull)	80mg
Decaffeinated coffee	5–15mg
Dark chocolate	80–160mg per 100g
Combination painkillers e.g. solpadeine	30mg per tablet

If you now look back at your diary, when do you take your caffeine and how much are you taking? The diary has asked you to mark how many caffeinated drinks you drink each day. You may well have heard about avoiding caffeine four to six hours before bedtime. This is because we know how long it takes your body to get rid of any chemical and this includes caffeine.

Caffeine has a half-life of between three to seven hours for most people. Earlier I explained that this is the time that it takes your body to get rid of half of the drug. However, this is not getting rid of all of it, just most of it. We are all different and some of us are more sensitive to the effects of caffeine than others. Therefore, we may still feel the effects for seven or eight hours. It is also important to think about how much caffeine we have had during the whole day. If you have had four cups of coffee at 4 p.m., you will still have between one and two full cups in your system at bedtime. This is why the diary needs to look at your whole twenty-four hours.

If you look at your diary and you see a pattern of several caffeinated drinks each day, then I would suggest either cutting down to no more than one cup in the morning or stopping altogether and just switching to drinks without caffeine in them. Beware, if you do decide to cut out caffeine that it is quite common to have a headache for three to four days after stopping. This is a mild withdrawal effect but it usually settles quickly. Could you continue to write down your caffeine drinks as you keep the diary over the next week?

Alcohol

Shakespeare wrote: 'Drink, sir, is a great provoker of three things . . . nose-painting, sleep, and urine. Lechery, sir, it provokes, and unprovokes; it provokes the desire, but it takes away the performance.'

Alcohol certainly does make you fall asleep a little quicker but the problem then comes in the second half of the night. The body breaks down alcohol very quickly and this means that it is out of your system in the second half of the night when it tends to cause both some vivid dreams and a lighter more broken sleep for most people. It also makes snoring worse and often makes you need to wake more to go to the toilet. So, using alcohol to get to sleep on a regular basis if you have insomnia is a really bad idea. It can also cause dependency and many other health problems. Count up how many drinks you have had in the week. It may be very little but if you are drinking more than three to four drinks close to bedtime, it would be a good idea to cut back to one or none while you are working through the therapy. It may be part of the reason that you are waking in the second half of the night.

Nicotine

Regular smokers often feel that cigarettes relax them and many people smoke close to bedtime as part of their bedtime routine. However, nicotine itself is a stimulant and also one that can make restless legs a little worse. If you do smoke and don't want to stop at the moment, make sure you have your last cigarette at least two hours before bedtime and avoid smoking in the night if you do wake up.

Exercise

There are lots of reasons to be physically fit but most people don't think of high-intensity exercise as a sleeping tablet. By high intensity, I mean exercise that really gets you out of breath and sweating. A simple guide would be whether or not you can talk easily in full sentences whilst exercising. If you are working hard at any type of exercise then you usually can't get to the end of the sentence that easily and you are sweating. These are simple measures of higher intensity levels. Look at your exercise levels in your diary over the last week – a lot of us plan to go to the gym or an exercise class a bit more often than we actually manage it! However, research has shown that high-intensity exercise is good for sleep and this includes those with chronic insomnia. The time of day and type of exercise do not seem to matter as long as you avoid exercise within the last two hours of the evening. Anything that gets you out of breath with your heart rate up for at least twenty to thirty minutes will have a good effect on your sleep. It helps you to both fall asleep quicker and to have deeper and more refreshing sleep. We should all be doing about 150 minutes of exercise a week. So, if you are not doing this, have a think about where this could fit into your day. Remember, it can be anything at all that gets your heart rate up and that suits you and your routines. You will feel both more alert after the exercise but are likely to sleep better overall. If you want additional information about how to measure exercise intensity there is more detail in the Resources section.

Getting ready for bed

The bedroom itself

This is something that some people can overcomplicate. In fact, the instructions around bed and the bedroom can be made very, very simple. I can name it in three.

Cool, dark and quiet

We have talked about how important light is in setting the body clock and sleep-wake cycle. We should all spend some time out of doors in natural light. In fact, the more the better. Making a point of being outside, even for your lunch break, as well as travelling to and from work/school will keep the clock set correctly. At the other end of the day, we want the bedroom to be dark; completely dark is best. Streetlights, children's night lights and many other things can make this difficult, but simple options to cut out the light include an eye mask or blackout blinds. Noise of course can disrupt anyone's sleep on occasion. So, if there is loud street noise then try to reduce this a little with some soft wax ear plugs. Research suggests that noise itself doesn't cause insomnia, which might surprise you. If you think back to a time when your sleep was better, you might remember that you were less sensitive to the odd sound at night. When you have insomnia, you tend to be much more alert and generally watchful. Your brain is more awake and so more tuned in to noise. This tuning in process is often the problem rather than the noise itself.

We should briefly tackle a few myths around the bedroom. Changing your mattress, your pillow or introducing herbal fragrances have really not been shown to make any difference to sleep (although the power of advertising may have convinced you otherwise). We know that if your bedroom is cool, dark and quiet, you are doing all the right things and it will be the other things that we teach you that will make the biggest difference to your sleep.

Having a clock in the bedroom is also a bad plan if you are sleeping badly. I have never yet had anyone tell me they felt better for looking at the clock at 2.34 a.m., waiting an eternity and then looking again only to see it is 2.37! In fact, people can start to count down the time remaining until the morning and describe anxiety increasing through the night with every hour that they see passing. So, get rid of the clock. Put it right out of sight and reach, ideally out of the bedroom entirely but at the door if you still need an alarm to get up. Make a positive decision to stop looking at it. This may seem a small thing but it can really help. And yes, this does include your smartphone if that has your clock on it. Your smartphone, laptop and tablet don't just have a clocks on them – they have most of your waking life on them with emails, photos, texts and work. I want your waking life out of the bedroom.

Do you go to sleep in your bedroom? This sounds like a silly question but some people use their bedroom for more than just sleep. When nights are long, when you stop thinking that you will fall asleep in bed, the relationship that you have with the bed and the bedroom can change. If you are awake for long periods, you might start to do things in bed that are part of your waking life: watching TV, reading, knitting or sudoku. This might seem like a good idea to decrease your levels of frustration but, in fact, this is simply reinforcing a pattern of bed being an awake place. Again, we can make this simple and say that the bedroom should be used for sleep only and none of your daytime activities. In particular, light sources such as laptops, phones and TV should be outside the bedroom.

I like the German word for bedroom, '*schlafzimmer*'; it literally means 'sleep room'. Make sure that your bedroom is a schlafzimmer and not a multipurpose room. When you read about Paul's story, our case history, you can see that he started to fall asleep on the sofa but often woke up with a headache or stiff neck. So, his bed place ended up being the sofa where he also watched TV. As the link between bed and sleep gets weaker it makes the problem worse (it is a good example of a perpetuating factor – something we might do because we are frustrated and often we think it might help but it becomes part of the problem). Can you look back again at the diagram on page 42.

A wind-down time before bed

If you think back to a time when you slept well, then you may not really have thought too hard about having a bedtime routine or doing things to wind down. You probably went fairly quickly to bed when you felt sleepy. It is worth thinking about what you do in the last thirty to sixty minutes before bedtime, particularly if you tend to work late or study or work at home. Working, thinking or worrying about work or the things we have to do the next day can add to a racing mind or a feeling of being too awake. Planning to put all work-related activities to one side, at least an hour before bed, is important. Some people find it helps to make a short list early in the evening of the key things they need to do the next day. Then that can be put to one side knowing the next day is planned and you can do something you enjoy before bedtime. That could be watching TV, reading, listening to music or doing crosswords. It really doesn't matter but it should be something that you find relaxing and that isn't really anything to do with your main daytime activities.

You may have thought about all of these lifestyle factors already, but use the table on page 77 to jot down any goals over the next five weeks for the lifestyle factors we have covered. You will be able to keep a check on yourself by continuing the sleep diary. It may be easiest to pick one lifestyle factor you are going to improve over the next week, for example getting back to the gym at least three to four times a week. Think ahead to exactly how you are going to do this. For example, it might be by planning to arrange to meet a friend after work to go to the gym together, or making sure that you take the stairs every single time at work rather than the lift. Then you can plan the days and the nights over the next week.

Summary of week 2 – sleep hygiene

Now, by looking at your diary, you can check the things that you do in the day that might affect your sleep and bedtime. You can make a plan to improve them over this next week and then keep these good habits going after this. This is your daytime life and habits. But you can also make sure that the bedroom itself is good for sleep, and that when you get ready for bed you have a plan to wind down and really put the day behind you.

Week 3 – Sleep scheduling – how to make a new sleep pattern

This is a big week for you and I am going to be honest, it may also feel tough and quite a challenge. This is because we are resetting your sleep patterns,

Lifestyle factor	Current (based on the diary)	Goal for next week	How you will do it
Cigarettes			
Exercise time			
Caffeine			
Alcohol			
Before bedtime			
Making the bedroom a sleep room			

so there are some big changes coming. There are some key changes that I want you to make over the next week. Two techniques called stimulus control and sleep restriction are going to give you some new sleep schedules. It can be difficult at first but we know that this is a really important part of the programme. Almost all of the people we treat tell us that this is helpful. Many years of sleep research has also shown that this is one of the most effective parts of the therapy and it is within the recommendations of all the current therapy manuals. You can also read through Poppy and Paul's stories (on pages 115 to 143) to see how they managed this part of the therapy.

First, I am going to help you to calculate your total sleep time. Let's have a look at the last seven days. The first thing that most people notice is that not every night is the same. To help I am going to show you Poppy's diary when she first came for treatment of her insomnia (pages 80–81).

Just as Poppy has, can you to add up the total amount of time you were asleep over the seven nights and divide by seven to get your average total sleep time (TST). Next, add up the hours you actually spent in bed and again divide by seven (time in bed – TIB). Then, we need to calculate your sleep efficiency which is TST/TIB. To take Poppy's as an example, her average total sleep time (TST) was 4 hours or 240 minutes. Her average time in bed (TIB) was 7.5 hours or 450 minutes. So sleep efficiency is TST/TIB, 240 minutes divided by 450 minutes. Poppy's sleep efficiency in Week 1 was 55 per cent.

Jot down the number in your sleep plan. So, what does that tell us? Well, it gives us a measure of how much of the night you actually spend asleep. To make sense of that number we need to think about what is normal. Not every night is the same but if you look over an average week, most adults will have a sleep efficiency of above 85 per cent. In other words, they spend most of the night in bed asleep. They might go to bed at about 11 p.m., fall asleep before 11.30 and wake up two or three times for a few minutes, but then fully wake up with the alarm at 7 a.m. People with insomnia usually have a lower sleep efficiency and are awake much more. It helps to start to measure your sleep and then we can see if the things that I will ask you to do are helping because we can measure your sleep again over the course of therapy. Remember what I said about the connection between bed and sleep? Well, if you spend more and more time in the bed awake then you lose that connection, frustration increases, how you feel and behave in bed tends to change and this makes insomnia even worse. Paul and Poppy both felt frustrated and angry about bad sleep. They were

Week 1 – Poppy

	p.m.							midnight / a.m.												noon / p.m.					
	6	7	8	9	10	11	12	1	2	3	4	5	6	7	8	9	10	11	12	1	2	3	4	5	6
Activities														C	C	C	C	C	M					M	
Sleep Time																									

LIGHTS OUT _9.45_ p.m.   TOTAL SLEEP TIME _5_ hrs

	p.m.							midnight / a.m.												noon / p.m.					
	6	7	8	9	10	11	12	1	2	3	4	5	6	7	8	9	10	11	12	1	2	3	4	5	6
Activities															C	C	C	C	M					M	
Sleep Time																									

LIGHTS OUT _10.00_ p.m.   TOTAL SLEEP TIME _5_ hrs

	p.m.							midnight / a.m.												noon / p.m.					
	6	7	8	9	10	11	12	1	2	3	4	5	6	7	8	9	10	11	12	1	2	3	4	5	6
Activities															C		C	C	M	M				M	
Sleep Time																									

LIGHTS OUT _10.00_ p.m.   TOTAL SLEEP TIME _3.5_ hrs

Chart 1

	p.m.							midnight / a.m.											noon / p.m.						
	6	7	8	9	10	11	12	1	2	3	4	5	6	7	8	9	10	11	12	1	2	3	4	5	6
Activities				→					T				↑			C	C		M					M	
Sleep Time																									

LIGHTS OUT *9.50* p.m. TOTAL SLEEP TIME *5.5* hrs

Chart 2

	p.m.							midnight / a.m.											noon / p.m.						
	6	7	8	9	10	11	12	1	2	3	4	5	6	7	8	9	10	11	12	1	2	3	4	5	6
Activities				A	→						T	↑		C	C					M					
Sleep Time																									

LIGHTS OUT *11.00* p.m. TOTAL SLEEP TIME *1.5* hrs

Chart 3

	p.m.							midnight / a.m.											noon / p.m.						
	6	7	8	9	10	11	12	1	2	3	4	5	6	7	8	9	10	11	12	1	2	3	4	5	6
Activities	M		→						T			↑		C				C	M						
Sleep Time																									

LIGHTS OUT *8.30* p.m. TOTAL SLEEP TIME *6* hrs

Chart 4

	p.m.							midnight / a.m.											noon / p.m.						
	6	7	8	9	10	11	12	1	2	3	4	5	6	7	8	9	10	11	12	1	2	3	4	5	6
Activities				→						↑→	↑				↑				M						
Sleep Time																									

LIGHTS OUT *10.10* p.m. TOTAL SLEEP TIME *2.5* hrs

starting to really **try** to fall asleep and this increased effort around bedtime can make things worse and not better, and then become part of the problem.

Strengthening the link between bed and sleep

I am going to tell you about two new techniques, called sleep restriction and stimulus control. Both of these techniques will really make you feel sleepy when you are in the bedroom. They are used to strengthen the association between bed and sleep and reset your sleep-wake system.

First, look at your diary, see whether you fall asleep quickly on most days or whether it takes you some time to fall asleep. Are you sleepy when you get into bed? This may sound like a silly question but many of my patients with insomnia say 'No' when I ask them this. When insomnia has been a big problem for months and years, people can really forget what it is like to feel sleepy close to bedtime. This can lead to getting into bed at different times or trying to go to bed earlier. Sometimes this is to try something different. People think that if they take an hour to fall asleep, getting into bed an hour earlier means that they will then fall asleep when they want to. In fact, this can make things worse rather than better.

It means you spend longer wide awake in bed so that the connection between bed and sleep is weakened or even lost. Bed becomes a place where you lie awake and feel frustrated rather than relax and fall asleep. As a result, some people start to dread going to bed, assuming that they won't sleep. 'Counting down the hours . . .', 'another bad night . . .' are all phrases I hear from my patients when they can't sleep. It all starts to make sleep and bedtime seem like an effort and something you are really focusing on.

So, we need to strengthen the connection between bed and sleep again, and stop you having long periods awake in the bedroom. Therefore, I am going to give you some very specific instructions.

1. *Only get into bed when you are sleepy – every single night.* Now this is different to feeling fatigued or bored. This means really, really sleepy, eyes gritty, yawning and waiting until that point every night. This may be later on some nights than others because we know that sleep is variable. When you slept well, you probably didn't get into bed at exactly the same time every night.

2. If you look at your diary, you will see nights when you got into bed but didn't sleep or times when you woke and lay awake for a long time. So, from now on we need a new rule. *If you do*

not fall asleep quickly then I want you to get up, go into another room and wait until you feel sleepy before heading back to bed. This is particularly important if you really feel wide awake and cross. Being cross and irritated makes your heart rate and adrenalin levels go up. This just makes you feel even more awake. So, we need to take that agitation out of the bedroom.

Now this might take some planning. You need to think about where you are going to go when you get up. Make sure it is somewhere warm, comfortable and with a low light level; ideally with a night light rather than the main room lights that are used in the day or early evening. Plan ahead before bedtime to leave nearby a book, newspaper or magazine, or have some music to listen to. I would prefer you to leave the screens and TV for the day to avoid the light levels that really wake your brain up. So, stick to reading, music, crossword puzzles or anything that you can do easily. Avoid anything too energetic that will really wake you up, like getting all the ironing done; leave these things for the daytime.

Now, if you do wake in the night you have a plan. Head back into the bedroom only when you feel really sleepy and your eyes are struggling to stay open. Then you are in bed when you are sleepy but up when you are not. This is sometimes called the quarter-hour rule – don't lie in bed, wide awake for more than about a quarter of an hour.

3. *Out of the bedroom during the day* – to strengthen the connection between the bed and sleep at night, you must avoid napping in bed during the day. Daytime is for being awake and if you sleep during the day, you will generally feel less sleepy at night. If you do really struggle to get through the day without napping, check you do not have another type of sleep disorder (see pages 48–55).

4. *Bed is for sleeping* – we covered this earlier in week 2 but to really reinforce the message, only sleep in bed. All of your other daytime activities, reading, TV, your phone and laptop should now be outside the bedroom. Look around and check you have done this. Sex is the exception to the rule: this tends to help sleep.

Sleep restriction

Now let's look at your sleep efficiency – good sleepers have high sleep efficiency and we want to create that for you. I want you to look at your total sleep time and work out the numbers of hours in bed that you would need to give you a sleep efficiency of over 85 per cent. Poppy's diary in the Case histories section (pages 122–31) is an example. To give her a sleep efficiency of 85 per cent, her time in bed would only be five and a half hours.

So, for the next week, I want to set some new bed and wake times for you. First of all, think about when you are going to get up. This is the fixed point in the day and I want you to keep it the same – seven days a week. Think of this as a line in the sand that you can't cross. This means that it is important to fix a time that suits you. When you slept well, when did you tend to wake? Try not to pick a time too late in the day. We know for most people over the age of twenty-five, this will be somewhere between 6 and 8 a.m.

You can see on page 128 that Poppy decided upon 6 a.m. Can you decide upon your wake time, write this down as your plan for the next week and really stick to it. Set an alarm clock if you need to for the weekends because this must be the same time on both weekdays and weekends. Good sleepers tend to have stable sleep patterns, so we want to give you this. Remember that you need to keep your body clock stable as well as your hours in bed.

Now we need to set your bedtime. If you want to sleep through the night, let's pick a bedtime that will help you to do this. You can see that Poppy set her bedtime for 00.30 a.m. Now, this may well seem late but the aim is to reset your sleep and take those gaps out of the night. This may seem tough but we know that this increases sleep efficiency and reduces frustration. It really strengthens the link between the bedroom and sleep. It also tends to make the sleep that you do have both deeper and more refreshing. It is also important to say that I am **not** telling you that this is your new pattern for ever. I promise it is just for a short time to reset the system. Think of it a bit like rebooting your computer to reset your sleep.

Getting into bed later can also take some planning. If other people are in the house then you may worry about keeping them awake if you are still up or disrupting their routines. You might have to think about things to do to pass the time without getting too bored. It might be the time to fold the washing or make the packed lunches, easy jobs that are not too strenuous and also not too stimulating. How about reading, listening to the radio, an audio book or a podcast? Watching TV is fine earlier on in the evening, but ideally cutting out TV and other screens or bright light after midnight is best. Knitting, crosswords, magazines, puzzles are all suggestions. Find something you would like to do but don't start baking cakes (then you will be stuck waiting for the oven timer) and if you are reading, try to avoid things related to work or the latest thriller. Short articles are better, which is why newspapers and magazines often work best. This may be a long time after your normal bedtime, so plan a couple of things to do so you can pass the time. **One important rule is not to make time in bed less than five hours when you are sleep restricting.** This ends up being too tough for most people and can cause trouble with daytime sleepiness or driving.

I am just going to summarise these new rules in the list below:

1. Get into bed at your new set bedtime and not any earlier, and make sure you are feeling really sleepy *(think about how you feel when your eyes are heavy – the nodding dog, rather than simply fatigued).*

2. If you do not fall asleep quickly or if you wake in the night and feel cross and too awake, get up and go into another room until you do feel sleepy *(think of this as a period of about quarter of an hour, or as long as it takes to feel like a long time, plan ahead for getting up if you need to).*

3. Get up every morning at your fixed wake time *(will you need to set an alarm? – make sure the clock is out of sight during the night but still within earshot – it can be by the door).*

4. Keep every day exactly the same for the next seven days *(the diary will help – you will be*

*filling it in every day so you can see your own
personal sleep plan).*

Can you now make your new sleep plan and write it
down in the box below. Make sure you write down
your own times based on the seven days of your
sleep diary.

My new set bedtime	
My times to get out of bed	
Where I will go if I wake and can't sleep	
What I will do if I wake to relax	

This is often the point in therapy when people start
to really worry and protest. Trust me, this is normal.
It feels quite brutal to take you out of the bedroom
but I did say that we were resetting the system.
Think of this as 'Control-Alt-Delete' for your night.

A complete overhaul will take all of those gaps out of the night. Then you can start to have several hours of more continuous sleep. I explained how the brain controls sleep – the longer you have been awake, the sleepier you get – the homeostat. This method helps to make bed somewhere you are sleepy again and strengthens the bed-sleep connection. Keeping everything the same, night and day, also keeps your body clock to a regular time. It is often very effective at breaking the cycle of associating the bedroom with being cross and wide awake.

Keep filling in the diary over the next seven days with your new plan and you will be able to monitor your progress. There is plenty of space in the diary in your book to jot down lights out, lights on, when you woke in the night and whether or not you got up.

Let's look at Poppy's diary (see page 130) as she goes through that first week of sleep scheduling. The first thing to spot is that lots of the gaps have gone from the night. Can you see that she is still waking, but the time awake is shorter and therefore her sleep efficiency has gone up. I think that her comments are honest and this is a tough process. She is starting to spend more time in bed asleep. Not every night is the same but instead of getting little bits of sleep, there are more times where she is sleeping for three to four hours at a time.

Summary of week 3 – a new sleep schedule

This week will now mark some big changes to your sleep schedule by teaching you how to work out your sleep efficiency and then restrict time in bed to make your sleep much more efficient without many gaps in the night. You will have a plan to be in the bedroom for less time and this will strengthen the association between bed and sleep. Please can you try your best to stick to this for the next week.

Week 4 – Adjusting the sleep schedule

'But I'm exhausted – now what?' Many patients say this to me after the first week of sleep restriction. It is really important to reassure you that I will not be keeping you permanently on this very short time in bed. Well done for getting to this stage and sticking with a tough treatment plan.

What is your sleep efficiency on the new schedule? You have now been doing this for a week. In the same way as before, work out your average over the seven days. Now you can see how important the diary really is to making all the week-by-week adjustments that you will need to improve your sleep. If your sleep efficiency is now 85 per cent or higher for one full week, you can increase your time in bed by fifteen minutes. Most people want to get into bed earlier, for example bed at 1.15 a.m. instead of bed at 1.30 a.m. I want you to be strict about this and only increase your time in bed if your sleep efficiency is high.

Each week from now on, increase your time in bed by fifteen minutes as long as your sleep efficiency stays high (above 85 per cent). You should still be falling asleep quickly on most of your nights. I still want to you to keep your wake time fixed. That anchor point to the first part of your day is important.

You might very well ask 'How long do I keep adding the fifteen minutes on to the time in bed?' Well, the easy answer is until you stop falling asleep quickly. Poppy's diary over week 4 shows you exactly how she adjusted her sleep schedule by getting into bed fifteen minutes earlier than in week 3.

Comments

'I took a break with Sam's rotten cold but back on track now.'

'My sleep efficiency is still high (89 per cent), so moving bedtime back by fifteen minutes, heading into bed when sleepy is easier now.

Now planning to keep wake time at 6 a.m. but with six hours in bed – luxury!'

Over this next week, please can you stick to my bossy rules about keeping a scheduled time in bed, and getting out of bed quickly if you are awake and cross. You are going to keep the diary going during this time as your own progress chart. This is where it can be really useful to remind yourself about some of your reasons for trying to improve your sleep. Going back to those initial goals you wrote down can be helpful if you need a reminder. You should be getting used to filling in the diary once a day, sticking to the good daytime habits we covered in week 2 and also the sleep scheduling from week 3.

Summary of week 4 – adjusting the sleep schedule

We have now covered a lot: in the first week you started to keep a sleep diary and then in the second

Week 4 – Poppy

Week 4 – Poppy

	6	7	8	9	10	11	12	1	2	3	4	5	6	7	8	9	10	11	12	1	2	3	4	5	6
	— p.m.						midnight / a.m.												noon / p.m.						
Activities		X	M									↑		C		C	C		M					M	
Sleep Time							→																		

LIGHTS OUT _00.15_ p.m.   TOTAL SLEEP TIME _5.5_ hrs

	6	7	8	9	10	11	12	1	2	3	4	5	6	7	8	9	10	11	12	1	2	3	4	5	6
Activities		X	M										↑	C			C	C		M					
Sleep Time							→																		

LIGHTS OUT _00.15_ p.m.   TOTAL SLEEP TIME _6_ hrs

	6	7	8	9	10	11	12	1	2	3	4	5	6	7	8	9	10	11	12	1	2	3	4	5	6
Activities		X						↑		→		↑						M						M	
Sleep Time							→																		

LIGHTS OUT _00.15_ p.m.   TOTAL SLEEP TIME _4.25_ hrs

Chart 1

	p.m.						midnight / a.m.												noon / p.m.						
	6	7	8	9	10	11	12	1	2	3	4	5	6	7	8	9	10	11	12	1	2	3	4	5	6
Activities		X												C	C				M						
Sleep Time							→					↑													

LIGHTS OUT *0.10* p.m.

TOTAL SLEEP TIME *5* hrs

Chart 2

	p.m.						midnight / a.m.												noon / p.m.						
	6	7	8	9	10	11	12	1	2	3	4	5	6	7	8	9	10	11	12	1	2	3	4	5	6
Activities		X												C						M					
Sleep Time							→						↑												

LIGHTS OUT *00.00* p.m.

TOTAL SLEEP TIME *6* hrs

Chart 3

	p.m.						midnight / a.m.												noon / p.m.						
	6	7	8	9	10	11	12	1	2	3	4	5	6	7	8	9	10	11	12	1	2	3	4	5	6
Activities	M	X												C				M							
Sleep Time							→						↑												

LIGHTS OUT *00.00* p.m.

TOTAL SLEEP TIME *5.5* hrs

Chart 4

	p.m.						midnight / a.m.												noon / p.m.						
	6	7	8	9	10	11	12	1	2	3	4	5	6	7	8	9	10	11	12	1	2	3	4	5	6
Activities		X												C						M					
Sleep Time							→						↑												

LIGHTS OUT *00.15* p.m.

TOTAL SLEEP TIME *5.5* hrs

week, the focus was on looking at your lifestyle and things you do by day and night that might affect sleep. In week 3, I told you about some tough new schedules to keep, and in the fourth week the focus was all about keeping those patterns and schedules really consistent. I want you to keep filling in the diary to make sure that the wake time stays the same and that you are not lying in the bedroom wide awake for any length of time over fifteen minutes. You can start to increase the time in bed a little if you are falling asleep quickly, but keeping the routine in week 4 very much the same as week 3 is important. This helps to maintain your new sleep schedule and improve your sleep. So keep to these rules over the next week.

Week 5 – How to slow down a racing mind and fall asleep more easily

During this week, I want to give you some simple techniques to help you fall asleep without getting out of bed. You might wonder why I didn't go through these a bit earlier? These techniques tend to work best **after** you have worked out your best sleep schedule. So over this next week, you might start to notice that sometimes you are waking but either the gaps in the night are shorter or you don't feel quite so cross. However, some people still feel very wide awake. If you look back at the diagram on page 42, you can see that these racing thoughts can be part of the cycle that maintains insomnia.

> Poppy – 'I don't have anything to worry about, I can feel sleepy sitting in front of the TV, really sleepy. Then I climb the stairs and get into bed and it is as if a light has switched on. Everything is going round in my head, I can't switch off, even though I feel exhausted.'

Many patients have told me over the years that they really struggle to switch off. They talk about a 'racing mind'. Do you feel as if your body is tired but your mind is still busy? If so, we are going to look at some techniques that will help you with this issue. There are things that you can do to slow down those racing thoughts and let your brain relax and sleep.

What sort of things are going round in your head when you are in bed? How do you feel in the bed? It might be that you are looking back over your day and planning ahead for the next one. Sometimes you start to tune in to your body, listening to your heart beat, starting to feel too hot with the duvet and just not comfortable. Do you feel tense or restless? Are you thinking about not sleeping or trying really hard **not** to think about not sleeping and what will happen after another bad night. Let's play a quick game – I want you to try really hard and, whatever you do, do **not** think about pink elephants. I bet there is an image of some kind of pinkish elephant sneaking into your head right now! So, however hard you try to put aside your last bad night, even thinking that you won't think about sleep can keep you awake.

> 'A ruffled mind makes a restless pillow.'
> – Charlotte Brontë

Maybe you are thinking about the next day, all the things you have to do or what went on during the day you have just had. If this happens, then I would like you to try this technique which is really a way of putting the day aside. This is a way of dealing with all of the planning and thoughts that go into your day a long time before your bedtime. Then you are not climbing into bed carrying those thoughts and worries with you.

Putting the day away

Set aside fifteen to twenty minutes in the early evening, at least two or three hours before your usual bedtime, for example at about 7 p.m. Make sure that you do this outside of the bedroom and in your normal waking space. This might be at the kitchen table or in the study if you have one. Get a notebook and pen ready or use your diary if you have one. You might want to use your phone or computer if you have an electronic calendar. Simply make a short list of the day that you have just had, what you did, the things that you managed to do and anything that you didn't do that bothered you.

Write down a short 'to do' list of the things you know that you need to do soon. This might be posting a bill, buying a present or a work deadline. For tomorrow, think about what you have to do at work or in the house. Write down a plan for the day including any jobs and an order in which to do them. Try to list two or three things. This is not a list for your whole month, just the next day, so keep the 'to do' list short and manageable. Check your diary so that you know that there are no surprises coming up. If there is anything that you are not sure about, make a note in your diary or on your phone to find out what you need to know and a time to do this (for example, before lunchtime). When you look down your list and feel in control of the day ahead, close the book and put it away. Get into the habit of putting the notebook in the same place. Now when it is coming close to bedtime, remember you have put the day to rest and then you will have dealt with some of the things that might be part of a racing mind.

Cognitive control techniques – slowing down a racing mind

You must have heard of the old story about counting sheep to get off to sleep? In fact this doesn't seem to work very well for people with insomnia. One reason might be that this is such a simple and boring thing to do that your mind can race off elsewhere again quite easily.

What I can give you is a different 'programme' to run. Again we are thinking about resetting the system. What you need is not sheep but an exercise that gives your mind something a bit more complicated to do, in fact quite a tiring task. Something that will be mentally complicated enough to stop the racing and help you drift off to sleep.

The first thing to say about these techniques is that they need a little practice and I am going to give you some choices. I want you to think of these techniques a little like a deck of cards where you might take a different card out of the pack on different nights. So, I will give you a visual task, but also a numbers task, a counting task and finally a word game. Before you take them into the bedroom, find a quiet time and a quiet place in the middle of the day when you can close your eyes and practise them for ten to fifteen minutes. You might find that you can do all of them equally easily or you might prefer the word game rather than the counting task. Different people think in different ways; this is why I am describing several different techniques. It honestly doesn't matter which one you prefer, just find the one that you can do best and concentrate on it. When you next climb into bed, start to run through your favourite one. All of these techniques are described as 'cognitive control' techniques. This simply means that they allow you to get more control over your thinking.

1. Visualisation

Think of a fruit that is easy to put into your mind in great detail, for example a banana. Think about it very carefully. Try to imagine the most perfect banana that you have ever seen, from the stalk all the way along the yellow lines, including the small dark marks. Once the picture is absolutely perfect, then slowly change the colour. Think of exactly the same piece of fruit, but as a blue colour. Again take your time to make the image as perfect as possible, as it would be in a painting. Think about how the brown stalk may now look blackish. When it is perfect, now change the colour again. You are unlikely to need to go through too many colours before you drift off to sleep.

2. Verbal techniques

Think about a category of objects, for example American states, different types of fruit or animals. Don't pick anything that is too close to something that you are emotionally involved in. For example, if you are a vet you might not want to choose animals. If you are using American states, think of the first American state that pops into your mind, for example Alabama. Now think of another state that begins with the last letter of this state (for example 'Arkansas'). Keep working through the sequence of words. It doesn't matter if you get them wrong and it doesn't matter if they are in any particular order. This is simply a way of creating a stream of words that doesn't have any particular emotion attached. It breaks the cycle of your mind fixing on any one thing. Switch categories if you are running out of ideas, but again most people find that they don't get through too many items before falling asleep.

3. Number techniques

Some people think in a more mathematical fashion. If you do, this technique may be worth trying. Start with the number one thousand and take away seven. Keep on going down: 993, 986, 979 and so on. Again, it doesn't matter if you make a mistake, but just keep working through the number sequence.

Try any of these techniques when you first get into bed and particularly if you feel as if your mind is starting to race or you are starting to feel agitated and bothered about not getting off to sleep. A lot of the things I am teaching you are deliberately designed to stop you from focusing on your sleep. We know that people with insomnia start to pay a lot of attention to their sleep. In fact this is very much part of the problem. So, all of the things I have been through here are things that distract you from your concerns about the night.

Progressive muscle relaxation

When you get into bed, do you feel relaxed or do you feel tense and tight? Some people struggle to relax. They tell me about muscle tension or 'tossing and turning'. You might have recognised this in the diagram we first went through on page 42.

One way to get round this is to learn how to control that muscle tension. It may seem strange trying to teach someone how to relax, but it is possible to teach these techniques. Relaxation is a skill which, just like any other, can be helped with practice; it really is like riding a bike. So I am going to teach you a very simple way to learn how to relax and let go as you are lying in bed. This involves tensing and then relaxing the main muscle groups in your body to decrease muscle tension, then breathing and heart rate.

It is best to practise this first outside the bedroom. Pick a time and a place where you won't be disturbed for at least fifteen to twenty minutes. Then, once you have practised the exercise a few times, you can start to use the technique in bed at night. The details of exactly how to do this are in the back of the book in the Resources section, page 160.

The words in the Resources section are the ones I use to teach my patients this technique and at the start, some people want either to record this themselves or play it from an audio file. There are some good audio files already out there and I have also given you details of one of these to listen to on page 163. However, over time, I would really like you to learn how to do this on your own so you can follow the sequence through in your mind.

Summary of week 5 – stopping your racing mind

This week gives you some different techniques to stop your mind racing and tension increasing when you are lying in bed. Remember, different techniques will suit different people and it is best to think of this book as a toolkit. You might use a different tool on a different night. So if you feel that your mind is racing, try the cognitive control techniques to give your mind another programme to run in order to slow down those thoughts. This makes it easier to drift off to sleep. Others are aware that they are physically tense and therefore will use the muscle relaxation techniques to control and then release that tension. Don't worry if some of the techniques don't seem to work for you or if you don't use all of them. Many people find one or two things that help them to fall off to sleep if they wake in the night or when they first get into bed. Planning for the next day well before bedtime can also help to make you feel more in control and so decrease the anxiety of a poor night ahead.

Week 6 – Putting it all together and keeping it together – The Relapse Prevention Toolkit

This final section is for people who have started to see an improvement in their sleep after working through the programme. For a start, if you are reading this with some sleep diaries that look better than before, then well done! It might be helpful to look back at your diaries to see what you have achieved in the last few weeks. Congratulations are in order; I know the therapy is hard work and often quite time consuming at the beginning. It is only by doing the things that I have asked you to do that your sleep has improved, so you have successfully helped your-self to sleep better.

The important next step is to work out how to keep progress going and make a plan to sleep well in the future. We can all have a bad night occasionally but I want to make sure you can cope with any problems that come up over the next few weeks. Research into insomnia has shown that people can often slowly improve over months by persisting with these techniques. Many people can feel quite positive at this stage but some people worry about what will happen when they stop CBTi, and in particular when they stop filling in sleep diaries. You might worry about slipping backwards. Therefore, even if things are better, I would really encourage you to read and work through this section as well.

Over the last few weeks, I have shown you how to measure your sleep using the sleep diary. Writing things down over the nights is usually your best guide to a good or bad night. So, at the end of the six-week programme, most people are waking up less, with fewer long gaps in the nights, so they have a higher sleep efficiency. Don't worry if this doesn't happen every night. Remember we are looking at the pattern over the weeks and not just over one or two days.

First of all, I just want to summarise what we have covered so far – these are the keys steps for beating insomnia.

1. Understanding your sleep

During sleep, we all wake and return to sleep about every ninety minutes and we all wake more as we get older. Natural light is vital to set the normal sleep-wake cycle. We all need to try and make sure we are outside for at least some part of every day. Good and bad sleepers will have the occasional bad night and this is normal.

We can think of insomnia as a bad habit tuning in to something that should be automatic and this can be corrected with simple techniques to reset your schedule and strengthen the bed-sleep connection. It is also important to take your focus away from the night and the bedroom – this helps to make sleep more automatic again.

2. Before bedtime

Look at any habits that affect sleep (caffeine, nicotine, alcohol) and make a plan to either cut down or stop.

Exercise is good for you – both your days and your nights will be better with moderate- to high-intensity exercise (out of breath is a good guide) put into each day for twenty to thirty minutes. If this has slipped because of your insomnia make sure it goes back in. Avoid exercise in the last two hours before bedtime.

Avoid daytime napping or dozing on the sofa – keep the night and the bedroom for sleep.

Stop any work at least ninety minutes before bed. Make a plan early evening for any jobs that need to be done the next day with a short list. Then you can put any daytime worries to one side well before bedtime.

3. At bedtime

Stay out of bed until you are really sleepy (not just tired) so you are most likely to fall asleep quickly. Set your alarm for the same time each morning, seven days a week.

The bedroom should be cool, dark and quiet. Bed is for sleep only, so the light should be turned off straight away with no clock visible.

If you can't sleep, if you fall asleep and then wake up, or if you feel wide awake and really cross for more than fifteen minutes, head out of the bedroom. Plan something quiet and relaxing to do in your living room, with low light levels, until you feel sleepy-tired again. Reading, music, puzzles, audiotapes or radio are all options but choose something that suits you. Repeat if necessary later in the night.

Practise the mental imagery techniques and number/letter games if you do wake in the night but feel relaxed. Practise your progressive muscle relaxation exercise if you feel tense or do not fall asleep quickly.

Planning for the future

Take a look at the sleep diaries that you have completed over the last few weeks. It is now quite helpful to have them all in front of you. Let's work out what has gone well and what might still be a problem. I know when I treat people that it is rarely all plain sailing and every one of my patients is different. Some find different techniques easier or harder, and of course some things are not relevant to them. If you have never smoked, you can ignore all the advice about cigarettes. Equally if you already go running every day, you can skip over (or jog past) all of the advice about exercise.

Write down in the space overleaf some of the things that you think helped and some of the things that did not suit you or didn't work.

Techniques that helped me	
Techniques that didn't help me	
Techniques that didn't apply to me	
Starting sleep efficiency	
Sleep efficiency now	

Now you can look at the things that worked for you. Looking at the recovery stories in Section 4 from Poppy and Paul will also show you that they used different bits of the CBT techniques to improve their sleep.

This is going to help you to understand which bits of the programme you are going to keep in place for the future to maintain good sleep patterns. Maybe exercise was the best thing for getting you off to sleep quickly and you can see this from your diary. If so, you know that it should be a part of your long-term routine. Maybe you could see that the cognitive control techniques and the alphabet game just suited you. It worked on most nights to help you drift off and stop the long gaps when you were awake. It might also make you really good at getting through dull car journeys with small children or boring meetings at work.

So when I am seeing people in the final week or so of therapy, they say things to me in clinic like:

> 'My sleep has been fine for a bit in the past and slipped, won't that happen now?'

> 'How will I know if it is getting worse again?'

> 'Now if I sleep badly then it feels like all the work was for nothing.'

> 'If I sleep badly for a few nights, do I have to do it all over again?'

> 'How long do I keep the diaries for?'

> 'If I am not keeping diaries, how do I know what my sleep plan is?'

So let's try and answer the last two questions about your sleep diaries and make a sleep plan moving forward. When you have got on top of your insomnia, you don't want things to slip backwards. So, you may still worry if you do stay awake a little longer or wake in the night for no particular reason. Remember that good sleepers will have a bad night from time to time and good sleepers also wake at night. The difference is they don't tend to worry about it quite as much or let it affect their daily routine. Brief waking is normal.

I have shown you how to monitor your sleep using a sleep diary. However, the programme you went through involved some really tough changes to your routine and I would not want you to continue those diaries long-term. There also comes a point where stopping filling in sleep diaries is a positive step because you can start to see that you are sleeping more nights than not and if you do wake, it is often not for long.

Most people who come to the sleep clinic fill in sleep diaries for us for about six weeks. After this, we ask them to stop filling in the diaries. By this time, you should be able to work out what time you are most comfortable waking up and getting up. So, I would like you to look at your diaries now and work out when you are most comfortable getting up in the morning? What time suited you best? So if it is seven in the morning then I would suggest you stick to this time. There will be some changes with holidays or other times when you might be up earlier or a bit later but for most days it should be fixed.

You also will now have thought about roughly how much time you usually spend asleep in bed. Keeping mostly to this time helps to keep your body clock and your homeostat regular. So that might be seven hours on most nights as it was for Poppy. We will all have occasional late nights but try to keep to a time in bed that suits. If you do sleep through an alarm because you are tired or have stayed up very late, then you may just need extra sleep. If you do have a bad night where you seem to be awake for a long time, it is best still to stay up until your normal bedtime on the next night and make sure that you feel sleepy before heading into bed.

There are some parts of the sleep plan that I would like you to stick with even if you are sleeping well, and this is part of keeping your sleep working well. Firstly, don't get into bed if you feel wide awake; this can quite quickly become part of the problem in insomnia and you have worked hard to feel sleepy again. Try to stick to listening to your body and getting into bed when you are really sleepy, not just bored or physically fatigued. Secondly, if you feel wide awake and are starting to feel cross about it, head out of the bedroom quickly and simply do something else. This can be reading or listening to music for a few minutes until you feel more relaxed and sleepy again. This rule is worth keeping going. Keep the agitation out of the bedroom. Keeping your waking life out of the bedroom is also important if possible. Remember the *schlafzimmer* – the sleep room. Keep the office work and your laptop and phone out of sight, ideally out of the room.

'If I sleep badly, do I have to do it all over again?'

The answer is that you can repeat the therapy and there is evidence to show that if it has worked before, it will work again, but ideally we want to spot the warning signs a long time before you need to start all over again. You will also know second time round which techniques were really effective by looking at the table on page 110.

'How will I know if it's getting worse again?'

If you are starting to feel frustrated about your sleep, measure your sleep efficiency with a sleep diary kept over a week. Has your sleep efficiency dropped below 85 per cent? Has it dropped to the level you measured before we started treatment? If so, go back to the key CBTi measures, all on page 82.

Section 4

RECOVERY STORIES

Case histories
Poppy's story

You met Poppy on page 27. Her GP diagnosed insomnia and gave her a self-help book to work through using some CBTi techniques. Now you can read her story in more detail and look at her sleep diary as she worked through the therapy. Her story may be different to yours but you can see some of the ups and downs of her treatment. Looking at her worksheets and sleep diary may be useful if you need prompts or help with filling in your own sheets.

I can't blame Sam because he is gorgeous, and Mum helps lots, but really the problems with sleep all seemed to start in those first few months after he was born. Of course you expect to be tired because all the books tell you that. But he seemed more colicky than all my friend's babies. He was up every hour and I was walking the floor with him like a bit of a zombie during my maternity leave. The health visitor helped a lot when she found out he had reflux and the GP gave him some medicine. After about six months he was only waking once a night. We had his first birthday party last week and he mostly falls asleep on his own and wakes at about six. I was so sleepy in those first few months but also really aware of having him in the house and needing to listen out for his crying. I just thought I would sleep through once he did, but now I am still waking. Sometimes I go in to check it wasn't him crying but mostly he is fast asleep. When I was on maternity leave I could nap in the day when he did, so the night wakenings didn't bother me too much.

I never thought I had a sleep problem before but it was Mum who reminded me that my childhood nickname was 'pin-drop Poppy'. I always woke up really easily, and ended up in my own bedroom because I said my sister's snoring kept me awake! I never really liked sleepovers with friends because I didn't sleep that well. I sometimes lay awake if I had to get something important sorted and I remember not sleeping a wink the night before the Ofsted inspectors came to the school where I work. Still, it never really bothered me until now.

It all seemed to get worse heading back to work. I was really looking forward to the school term. We had a new form teacher and nursery was all sorted for Sam, but it was a different routine. I wanted to spend the evenings with him, so I tended to keep the housework until later in the evenings. Sometimes getting into bed I would still be thinking about the next day at school and then I couldn't sleep although I felt really weary. Sometimes it seemed like such a long time. Mike always falls asleep so easily, so I didn't want to get up and disturb him or Sam. Lying there started to really get to me and then I read an article in the newspaper about how important sleep is for your health and how it helps your memory. That night, I decided to go to bed really early to get eight hours sleep and it was a disaster! I got into bed at 7.30 p.m., straight after Sam but I felt really rest-less and a bit cross. I tried counting sheep, which didn't work at all.

I could manage with the odd bad night but it seemed to get worse and worse over the first school term. I started to get quite bothered walking to-wards the bedroom. I have never really been aware of my heart beat but lying in bed I could count it and it seemed far too fast. I wondered if there was something wrong with me and not sleeping was a warning sign.

That was the first time I went to the doctor. He was nice but he examined me quite quickly. He took some blood tests and told me that lots of young mums have broken nights but it tends to settle, so not to worry. He also said not to drink coffee or smoke before bedtime, but I don't drink any coffee anyway; it gives me heartburn. The blood tests were normal but I was a bit disappointed, which sounds silly. I thought if I was anaemic or something then treatment would make me sleep better.

Now I seemed stuck in a pattern. Sam went to bed and then I felt I had lots to do but was just so tired I often couldn't keep my eyes open on the sofa. Mike would tell me just to go to bed and get a good night's sleep. That would just make me cross and I would snap at him. Fine for him to say – just snoring away, it was like sleeping next to a grizzly bear! But when I went into the bedroom, it felt as if someone had switched a light on and I felt all restless and tense. Sometimes I would drift off but then jolt awake again in the night and it was only an hour or so later. I used to count down until the morning. Sometimes I got up and just put the lights on downstairs and gave up trying to sleep. Once I did all the ironing in the house, even Sam's sleepysuits. Every now and then I would crash and have five or six hours and I felt so much better in the mornings, but that hardly ever happened after a few months. I tried everything, new mattresses and going into the spare room in case it was Mike's snoring waking me. I plagued the life out of our local pharmacist trying every herbal remedy for sleep she had. None of it worked and when I went back the GP I was really feeling desperate. Not sleeping was affecting everything.

It was a different doctor, she was nice, really sympathetic. I think it helped that she had young children too. She spent a bit of time talking about my mood and asking if I was anxious. I didn't think I was, only bothered because I couldn't sleep. She talked about depression but agreed with me that this wasn't really the problem. She also asked me questions about sleepiness during the day and went through some different score sheets with me. I didn't really sleep during the day, I didn't sleep at all – that was the problem! So she said I had insomnia and she talked about sleeping tablets. She said she could give me them for two weeks but they often caused side effects. She also said that there was a different treatment, a type of CBT that took a bit longer but was often good at making people less bothered about their sleep. She used the phrase Talking Therapies and I didn't really know what that meant.

She said that she had a self-help book that one of her other patients had used to improve their sleep and that patient had been sleeping badly for longer than me – five years. I did say that I had already tried everything to help myself; that was why I wanted help. In fact, I really felt quite sceptical about a book being any use at all. She asked me if I had ever written down my sleep patterns in a diary and I hadn't, so she asked me at least to read the book and go through the first few chapters. She made another appointment to see me in four weeks and said she could talk again about sleeping tablets then. She also showed me a recent newspaper article where a psychologist was explaining that not many people know about this type of CBT but there was lots of research to show it helped. When I got home I started the book there and then before Sam got back from nursery. I thought that if I read it, I could at least tell the GP that I had tried everything before asking for some sleeping tablets.

I was surprised at first to find out how much I didn't know about sleep itself. Some of it was really interesting, especially the bit about waking at night and the different sleep stages. I also read up all the bits about the other sleep problems but none of those problems sounded like mine. I began to think the GP was right and it was all insomnia. The bit about adrenalin keeping you awake certainly made sense.

Over the next week I started to fill in the sleep diary. At first I really struggled with the very first instruction of taking the clock out of the bedroom. How could I fill in the diary without a clock? But Mike read through it with me and told me just to guess. He said he never looked at the clock. He just got up when the alarm went, so I put the clock outside the bedroom door. Anyway, after a few days I could start to see some patterns. Writing it down made me realise how long I was lying awake but also that I was getting some sleep on most nights. Only about three or four hours a night but I was getting some. Also, I could see that Sunday night was really bad. The diary asked me about exercise and I realised that I didn't do anything that week and I thought back to the Pilates classes I had time for before Sam came along. I never really thought about the things in the day that made my sleep worse. I realised I thought about it the other way round and blamed a bad night as the reason I didn't go to the gym. There were some things I read about in the sleep hygiene section that didn't apply to me, although we worked out that Mike's snoring is definitely worse after his Saturday-night beer, see overleaf. When I looked up how much caffeine was in my weak tea, I thought it wasn't worth me stopping it but I decided not to have any after 2 p.m. just to be sure.

Week 1 – Poppy

	p.m.						midnight / a.m.												noon / p.m.					
	6	7	8	9	10	11	12	1	2	3	4	5	6	7	8	9	10	11	12	1	2	3	4	5	6
Activities				↓										C	C	C	C	C	M					M	
Sleep Time													↑												

LIGHTS OUT _9.45_ p.m.

TOTAL SLEEP TIME _5_ hrs

	p.m.						midnight / a.m.												noon / p.m.					
	6	7	8	9	10	11	12	1	2	3	4	5	6	7	8	9	10	11	12	1	2	3	4	5	6
Activities					↓									C	C	C	C		M					M	
Sleep Time													↑												

LIGHTS OUT _10.00_ p.m.

TOTAL SLEEP TIME _5_ hrs

	p.m.						midnight / a.m.												noon / p.m.					
	6	7	8	9	10	11	12	1	2	3	4	5	6	7	8	9	10	11	12	1	2	3	4	5	6
Activities					↓		↕	↑						C	C			C	M					M	
Sleep Time													↑												

LIGHTS OUT _10.00_ p.m.

TOTAL SLEEP TIME _3.5_ hrs

Chart 1

	p.m.						midnight / a.m.												noon / p.m.					
---	6	7	8	9	10	11	12	1	2	3	4	5	6	7	8	9	10	11	12	1	2	3	4	5	6
Activities				→					T								C	C	M					M	
Sleep Time												←													

LIGHTS OUT *9.50* p.m.

TOTAL SLEEP TIME *5.5* hrs

Chart 2

	p.m.						midnight / a.m.												noon / p.m.					
---	6	7	8	9	10	11	12	1	2	3	4	5	6	7	8	9	10	11	12	1	2	3	4	5	6
Activities				A							T			C	C				M						
Sleep Time						→						←													

LIGHTS OUT *11.00* p.m.

TOTAL SLEEP TIME *1.15* hrs

Chart 3

	p.m.						midnight / a.m.												noon / p.m.					
---	6	7	8	9	10	11	12	1	2	3	4	5	6	7	8	9	10	11	12	1	2	3	4	5	6
Activities	M		→											C			C	C	M						
Sleep Time												←													

LIGHTS OUT *8.30* p.m.

TOTAL SLEEP TIME *6* hrs

Chart 4

	p.m.						midnight / a.m.												noon / p.m.					
---	6	7	8	9	10	11	12	1	2	3	4	5	6	7	8	9	10	11	12	1	2	3	4	5	6
Activities					→				t	←→					←				M						
Sleep Time												─													

LIGHTS OUT *10.10* p.m.

TOTAL SLEEP TIME *2.5* hrs

I decided to start doing some more exercise again. I didn't want to go back to the gym as I thought it would take too much time. I found an exercise video on the internet which only took twenty minutes and did that straight after Sam had gone to bed. I was hopeless at all the exercises I had previously been good at but I noticed that I had a bit more energy to get my work done before bedtime. I filled in the diaries for another week to see if exercise alone would fix it all. My sleep was a bit better but I could still see the big gaps during the night.

Week 2 – Poppy

Chart 1

	p.m.							midnight / a.m.												noon / p.m.					
	6	7	8	9	10	11	12	1	2	3	4	5	6	7	8	9	10	11	12	1	2	3	4	5	6
Activities		X	M												C	C	C		M					M	
Sleep Time				→																					

LIGHTS OUT 10.00 p.m.

TOTAL SLEEP TIME 4.5 hrs

Chart 2

	6	7	8	9	10	11	12	1	2	3	4	5	6	7	8	9	10	11	12	1	2	3	4	5	6
Activities		X	M											C		C	C		M					M	
Sleep Time				→																					

LIGHTS OUT 9.45 p.m.

TOTAL SLEEP TIME 4 hrs

Chart 3

	6	7	8	9	10	11	12	1	2	3	4	5	6	7	8	9	10	11	12	1	2	3	4	5	6
Activities		X																M						M	
Sleep Time						→																			

LIGHTS OUT 11.00 p.m.

TOTAL SLEEP TIME 5 hrs

Chart 1

	6	7	8	9	10	11	12	1	2	3	4	5	6	7	8	9	10	11	12	1	2	3	4	5	6
	p.m.						midnight / a.m.												noon / p.m.						
Activities		X												C			C		M					M	
Sleep Time				↓					↑	→			↑												

LIGHTS OUT *10.00* p.m.   TOTAL SLEEP TIME *5.5* hrs

Chart 2

	6	7	8	9	10	11	12	1	2	3	4	5	6	7	8	9	10	11	12	1	2	3	4	5	6
Activities		X												C					M					M	
Sleep Time				↓							↑														

LIGHTS OUT *9.50* p.m.   TOTAL SLEEP TIME *5.5* hrs

Chart 3

	6	7	8	9	10	11	12	1	2	3	4	5	6	7	8	9	10	11	12	1	2	3	4	5	6
Activities		X												C				M						M	
Sleep Time					↓							↑													

LIGHTS OUT *10.00* p.m.   TOTAL SLEEP TIME *4.5* hrs

Chart 4

	6	7	8	9	10	11	12	1	2	3	4	5	6	7	8	9	10	11	12	1	2	3	4	5	6
Activities		X												C						M					M
Sleep Time					↓						↑														

LIGHTS OUT *10.00* p.m.   TOTAL SLEEP TIME *4.5* hrs

Poppy's sleep efficiency at week 2

Average time asleep at night over the seven days is her total sleep time or TST for short – 4.5 hours or 270 minutes.

Average time in bed (or TIB for short) 8 hours or 480 minutes.

So sleep efficiency is TST/TIB.

For Poppy this is 270 minutes/480 minutes = 56 per cent.

It was quite fiddly working out the sleep efficiency after the second week. In fact, Mike and I argued about it. Once we added it all up in minutes it was easier. In the end we agreed it was 56 per cent.

When I read the part about decreasing my time in bed I felt really bothered – if I felt this bad on three or four hours a night, what would happen if I didn't sleep at all? I wasn't sure I could manage it. Mike wasn't sure either. He was already getting the brunt of my bad moods after bad nights, but I went for it with only five and a half hours in the bed. Mum said she would give me extra help with Sam if I needed it and I decided to go into the spare room for those two weeks to avoid disturbing Mike coming to bed after midnight. I made getting up at 6 a.m. the plan because that's when Sam usually wakes up. Mike loved that – it meant he got weekends off from Sam duty!

Well it was brutal for the first few days, staying up when I really craved sleep. One night I was really struggling to stay awake on the sofa. Amazingly, looking at my diary, it helped me to fall asleep. I started to feel a bit more like I had when Sam was tiny and I napped during the day. Instead of just being bone weary, I was struggling to keep my eyes open. I knew what the book meant by sleepy-tired. One day I got up at 6 a.m. and felt so sleepy, I was a bit bothered about driving but Mike gave me a lift to school and then once I was in the classroom I felt brighter again. I couldn't really believe the diaries when I looked at them. Five hours every night apart from Sunday, I think that was work Monday morning (page 130). Mike was a star and he kept reminding me to do the exercises. One day I missed them out but mostly we managed to stick to the plan between us.

Week 3 – Poppy

	p.m.						midnight / a.m.													noon / p.m.					
	6	7	8	9	10	11	12	1	2	3	4	5	6	7	8	9	10	11	12	1	2	3	4	5	6
Activities		X	M												C	C	C		M					M	
Sleep Time																									

LIGHTS OUT _00.30_ p.m.

TOTAL SLEEP TIME _5.5_ hrs

	p.m.						midnight / a.m.													noon / p.m.					
	6	7	8	9	10	11	12	1	2	3	4	5	6	7	8	9	10	11	12	1	2	3	4	5	6
Activities		X	M											C	C	C	C		M						
Sleep Time																									

LIGHTS OUT _00.30_ p.m.

TOTAL SLEEP TIME _5.5_ hrs

	p.m.						midnight / a.m.													noon / p.m.					
	6	7	8	9	10	11	12	1	2	3	4	5	6	7	8	9	10	11	12	1	2	3	4	5	6
Activities		X												C				M						M	
Sleep Time																									

LIGHTS OUT _00.15_ p.m.

TOTAL SLEEP TIME _5_ hrs

	p.m.						midnight / a.m.													noon / p.m.					
	6	7	8	9	10	11	12	1	2	3	4	5	6	7	8	9	10	11	12	1	2	3	4	5	6
Activities		X												C	C				M						
Sleep Time							→					←													

LIGHTS OUT _00.40_ p.m. TOTAL SLEEP TIME _5.5_ hrs

	p.m.						midnight / a.m.													noon / p.m.					
	6	7	8	9	10	11	12	1	2	3	4	5	6	7	8	9	10	11	12	1	2	3	4	5	6
Activities														C					M					M	
Sleep Time							→		←	→↓		←													

LIGHTS OUT _00.30_ p.m. TOTAL SLEEP TIME _3.15_ hrs

	p.m.						midnight / a.m.													noon / p.m.					
	6	7	8	9	10	11	12	1	2	3	4	5	6	7	8	9	10	11	12	1	2	3	4	5	6
Activities		X												C											
Sleep Time							→					←													

LIGHTS OUT _00.25_ p.m. TOTAL SLEEP TIME _6_ hrs

	p.m.						midnight / a.m.													noon / p.m.					
	6	7	8	9	10	11	12	1	2	3	4	5	6	7	8	9	10	11	12	1	2	3	4	5	6
Activities		X												C						M					
Sleep Time							→					←													

LIGHTS OUT _00.30_ p.m. TOTAL SLEEP TIME _5.5_ hrs

Comments and Poppy's sleep efficiency week 3

The sleep plan was 5.5 hours in bed.

Bed at 00.30 p.m. and fixed wake time at 6 a.m.

Total sleep time average over seven days is 5 hours or 300 minutes.

Time in bed 5.5 hours or 330 minutes.

Sleep efficiency 300/330 = 91 per cent.

Success! Over 85 per cent sleep efficiency, so for week 4, bedtime moved back to 00.15 p.m. but wake time still fixed at 6 a.m. Aiming for 5 hours 45 minutes in bed.

Having said that I was really starting to struggle to stay awake in the evenings, Mike was nudging me when I was on the sofa. I often had to stand up and walk around to stop myself dozing after midnight, so by week 4 when I started to go into bed earlier it seemed a godsend. I decided to keep the 6 a.m. starts. I realised that even at weekends, I was waiting for Sam to get up and that quiet time in the morning before Mike woke was quite nice. I got to six hours in bed and then Sam had a cold and gave it to me and everything seemed to go wrong for a few days. When I lay down, my head was full and sore and I had a bit of a temperature. I read the book and stopped the diaries until both Sam and I stopped sniffling, then I started again. I started to try the mind game and imagery exercises. I was no good at the numbers one (maths was never my best subject at school) but I quite liked making the pictures. That did seem to help if I woke in the night. I read all about getting out of bed if I was cross, but the diaries showed me that I didn't really spend that long awake any more (weeks 4 and 5).

By the time I came to the end of the programme I started to worry about slipping back again. I went through the last section and it felt like other people had all of the same worries, which helped a bit. I made a plan and stuck it on the fridge for 6 a.m. wake-ups (until Sam is a teenager??) and bed between 11.30 and 12 p.m. On the nights I missed my exercises, it didn't really seem to make a big difference to how many hours I spent in bed, but I just felt a bit sluggish so I kept those in. When I first saw the GP after four weeks, she said I looked tired but happier. When she saw me again after eight weeks, we both agreed I didn't need sleeping tablets. I am so glad I took the plunge and started the therapy. I don't think I will ever be a deep sleeper like Mike (he is now only allowed his beer at lunch and that has stopped the snoring), but now at least a few pins can drop before I wake!

Week 5 – Poppy

Chart 1

	p.m. 6	7	8	9	10	11	12	a.m. 1	2	3	4	5	6	7	8	9	10	11	12	p.m. 1	2	3	4	5	6
Activities		X	M												C	C	C		M						M
Sleep Time							↓	━	━	━	━	━	↑												

LIGHTS OUT _00.00_ p.m.

TOTAL SLEEP TIME _5.5_ hrs

Chart 2

	p.m. 6	7	8	9	10	11	12	a.m. 1	2	3	4	5	6	7	8	9	10	11	12	p.m. 1	2	3	4	5	6
Activities		X	M											C			C		M						
Sleep Time							↓	━	━	━	━	━	↑												

LIGHTS OUT _00.00_ p.m.

TOTAL SLEEP TIME _5_ hrs

Chart 3

	p.m. 6	7	8	9	10	11	12	a.m. 1	2	3	4	5	6	7	8	9	10	11	12	p.m. 1	2	3	4	5	6
Activities		X																M							M
Sleep Time							↓	━	━	━	━	━	↑												

LIGHTS OUT _00.00_ p.m.

TOTAL SLEEP TIME _4.75_ hrs

Chart 1

	p.m.						midnight / a.m.												noon / p.m.					
	6	7	8	9	10	11	12	1	2	3	4	5	6	7	8	9	10	11	12	1	2	3	4	5	6
Activities		X												C			C		M						
Sleep Time						→							↑												

LIGHTS OUT *11.45* p.m.

TOTAL SLEEP TIME *6* hrs

Chart 2

	p.m.						midnight / a.m.												noon / p.m.					
	6	7	8	9	10	11	12	1	2	3	4	5	6	7	8	9	10	11	12	1	2	3	4	5	6
Activities		X												C					M						
Sleep Time						→							↑												

LIGHTS OUT *11.45* p.m.

TOTAL SLEEP TIME *6.15* hrs

Chart 3

	p.m.						midnight / a.m.												noon / p.m.					
	6	7	8	9	10	11	12	1	2	3	4	5	6	7	8	9	10	11	12	1	2	3	4	5	6
Activities		X												C											
Sleep Time						→							↑												

LIGHTS OUT *11.45* p.m.

TOTAL SLEEP TIME *6* hrs

Chart 4

	p.m.						midnight / a.m.												noon / p.m.					
	6	7	8	9	10	11	12	1	2	3	4	5	6	7	8	9	10	11	12	1	2	3	4	5	6
Activities		X												C					M						
Sleep Time						→							↑												

LIGHTS OUT *11.30* p.m.

TOTAL SLEEP TIME *6* hrs

Week 6 – Poppy

	6	7	8	9	10	11	12	1	2	3	4	5	6	7	8	9	10	11	12	1	2	3	4	5	6
	p.m.						midnight / a.m.													noon / p.m.					
Activities		X	M											C	C		C		M						M
Sleep Time					→		━	━	━	━	━	━	←												

LIGHTS OUT *11.30* p.m.

TOTAL SLEEP TIME *6* hrs

	6	7	8	9	10	11	12	1	2	3	4	5	6	7	8	9	10	11	12	1	2	3	4	5	6
Activities		X	M											C			C		M						
Sleep Time					→		━	━	━	━	━	━	←												

LIGHTS OUT *11.30* p.m.

TOTAL SLEEP TIME *6.15* hrs

	6	7	8	9	10	11	12	1	2	3	4	5	6	7	8	9	10	11	12	1	2	3	4	5	6
Activities		X																	M						M
Sleep Time						→	━	━	━	━	━	━	←												

LIGHTS OUT *11.30* p.m.

TOTAL SLEEP TIME *6* hrs

Chart 1

	_	_	_	_	_	_	midnight / a.m.												noon / p.m.						
	6	7	8	9	10	11	12	1	2	3	4	5	6	7	8	9	10	11	12	1	2	3	4	5	6
Activities		X			C									C					M						
Sleep Time						↑							↑												

LIGHTS OUT *11.15* p.m.   TOTAL SLEEP TIME *5* hrs

Chart 2

	6	7	8	9	10	11	12	1	2	3	4	5	6	7	8	9	10	11	12	1	2	3	4	5	6
Activities		X					M							C											M
Sleep Time						↑							↑												

LIGHTS OUT *11.15* p.m.   TOTAL SLEEP TIME *5.5* hrs

Chart 3

	6	7	8	9	10	11	12	1	2	3	4	5	6	7	8	9	10	11	12	1	2	3	4	5	6
Activities		X												C											
Sleep Time						↑							↑												

LIGHTS OUT *11.15* p.m.   TOTAL SLEEP TIME *5.5* hrs

Chart 4

	6	7	8	9	10	11	12	1	2	3	4	5	6	7	8	9	10	11	12	1	2	3	4	5	6
Activities		X						M						C											
Sleep Time						↑							↑												

LIGHTS OUT *11.15* p.m.   TOTAL SLEEP TIME *6* hrs

Techniques that helped me	Exercise – back to pilates at least 3 times a week, wake time at 6, bed when sleepy
Techniques that didn't help me	Didn't like the muscle relaxation
Techniques that didn't apply to me	Don't smoke and no TV/lights in the bedroom
Starting sleep efficiency	56 per cent
Sleep efficiency now	85 per cent

Comments – 'sticking to 6 seems to work, I am almost always awake waiting for Sam to wake anyway. I haven't had to get out of bed for a while, I do the "making a picture" or the alphabet game if I wake and I hardly ever get to the end so I must be falling asleep. I know I still wake but that horrible feeling when I was climbing the stairs has gone. Time to stop the diaries I think.'

Paul's story

I could always sleep really well, hotels, airplanes, car passenger, you name it. If I was given the chance I could snooze and I loved my bed. Regular life, a bit of Saturday football and the gym in the week until that stupid flu bug. I know women say 'man flu' but this was the full monty, absolutely flat out with a head on fire and all of us vomiting. That's two children under six and two adults off work and school for a full two weeks. I felt really wiped out and couldn't even think about the gym for a week after that. I was still taking nasal decongestant back at work for a bit.

Then, the first night without a temperature I just couldn't sleep. It was really odd. It just doesn't usually happen. I remember feeling cross and a bit puzzled as Susan was sleeping next to me. I just thought it would settle but it was on my mind a bit the next night and then I was trying not to think about it. Maybe that made it worse because then I seemed to lie there for ages. When the alarm did go,

I felt like I had barely slept at all and struggled to get up. Two more nights and I was sick of it and went out of the bedroom because I was starting to annoy Susan. I put on the TV and next thing I knew it was morning and the kids were waking me with a stiff neck from sleeping on the sofa. I had a headache. Susan blamed the brandy I had taken to get off to sleep, but I thought it was not sleeping. There was a big meeting at work with the regional sales team that day. I know I was under par and performing badly because the boss gave me a hard time about it afterwards.

Then it just all seemed to spiral a bit. I tried going back to bed as normal but I would just lie there getting cross and bothered. Then my neck and head seemed to hurt. I always knew that a drink at the weekend made me fall asleep, so it seemed logical just to have brandy at night, but then that stopped working. Over the next few weeks, going to sleep suddenly seemed like this big deal. It seemed a really stupid thing to have a problem with. I had nothing to worry about, I went to the GP thinking it was the flu hanging around and asked for some blood tests. I thought maybe some antibiotics or something could just make me feel normal again. The GP didn't do any tests but just told me to forget about it and that everything would settle.

Well it didn't. I was getting grumpy with Susan, in fact I was getting cross with everyone, particularly all those people who could sleep. For some reason, everyone seemed to sleep well but me. I had never even noticed adverts for mattresses and pillows before. Now they seemed to be everywhere, smug snoozing people on pictures. It was just rubbing it in.

Getting into bed was the worst; I just knew I wouldn't sleep, so I stopped trying because Susan and I started to argue every night about it. I went downstairs and thought that using the TV to fall asleep would be best because then I wouldn't be stressing about not sleeping.

It did work but my headaches got worse. In fact, that was why I ended up going back to the GP. I really thought that there must be something wrong. It was almost a year after the flu when I ended up demanding blood tests and some kind of scan. I thought that I was going to lose my job or not be safe to drive. I just needed one good night of sleep.

The GP did listen this time. She examined me, looked in my eyes, did some blood tests and gave me a leaflet about sleep. Some of the things that it said were bad for sleep were things I knew I did. When I went again, I told the GP I couldn't go back into the bedroom or Susan would just be really sick of me. The GP told me about something called Talking

Therapies and said that she was going to refer me to someone who could help. I was a bit dubious until she said that it was a bit like a self-help group to stop smoking, or a personal trainer.

It took a few weeks but a lady called Rekke rang me. She was really straightforward, quite businesslike really. She just went through some questions and, for the first time, I was talking to someone who sounded like she knew what she was talking about. It was a real relief just to go through it in detail. She asked quite a lot of questions and then she gave me some charts to fill in. She had already picked up that I was drinking quite a lot. I explained that it was the only thing that got me off to sleep but she told me how alcohol actually made your sleep worse. I didn't really know that. I started to see that some of how I felt during the day was due to too much booze. We made a plan to cut that right down and then when I brought back the diaries, she picked up on all the agitation just before bed.

First of all she banned the sofa! It seems like such a small thing – where you sleep – but it took some major furniture shifting. I realised that I hadn't slept with Susan for weeks and so we agreed to try the spare room. It was full of junk and boxes so I had to clear that one weekend. Funnily enough I did sleep better then. After that the TV went off after midnight and she explained all about light and dark affecting your sleep.

Over the next few weeks she made me really look at all the things I was doing. I thought it was helping but it was actually making it worse. The biggest help were the things that she gave me to get me off to sleep. First some relaxation tricks that felt a bit like things I might do at the gym. Then some techniques to stop me getting really wound up when I was lying in bed. I also started to go back to the gym. I didn't really think that made much difference to sleep, but it was good to see friends again and it made me more relaxed during the day.

Writing it down was the big difference. When I thought things were not working or if I had a bad night, Rekke showed me my sleep diaries over time. She made me realise that lots of my friends and even Susan slept badly sometimes. After a couple of months, I was falling asleep much quicker and even when I didn't, I just wasn't getting so wound up about it. The booze was back to weekends only and the boss was off my back. I started to head back into the bedroom with Susan, which was really nice. We agreed that I could always head to the spare room if I couldn't sleep, but mostly I didn't need to. I stopped seeing Rekke but she said I could get back in touch if I needed to. Fingers crossed so far, I haven't needed to.

RESOURCES

SLEEP DIARY

Date started_____

Day of Week_____

Instructions:

- Leave the diary near your bedside

- Fill out this chart each morning but not during the night

- Mark your diary in the following way:

ACTIVITIES

A	–	each alcoholic drink
C	–	each caffeinated drink, including coffee, tea, chocolate, cola
P	–	every time you take a sleeping pill
M	–	meals
S	–	snacks
X	–	exercise
T	–	use of toilet during sleep-time
N	–	noise that disturbs your sleep
W	–	time of wake-up alarm (if any)

SLEEP TIME (including naps)

↓	–	mark with a 'down' arrow each time you got into bed
↑	–	mark with an 'up' arrow each time you got out of bed
|	–	mark with a line the time you began and the time you ended your sleep; then join the line to indicate sleep periods
|	–	mark with a line the time you began and the time you ended any naps, either in the chair or in bed; then join up lines with a broken line to indicate nap periods

Note down any events that influenced your sleep

Example

	p.m.					midnight / a.m.											noon / p.m.						
	6	7	8	9	10	11	12	1	2	3	4	5	6	7	8	9	10	11	12	1	2	3	4	5	6
Activities	A	A	A		S						T				W	S			M		S		M		
Sleep Time																									

LIGHTS OUT __12.30__ p.m.

TOTAL SLEEP TIME __6__ hrs

Week 1

		p.m.						midnight / a.m.												noon / p.m.					
	6	7	8	9	10	11	12	1	2	3	4	5	6	7	8	9	10	11	12	1	2	3	4	5	6
Activities																									
Sleep Time																									

LIGHTS OUT_____ a.m. / p.m.   TOTAL SLEEP TIME_____ hrs

		p.m.						midnight / a.m.												noon / p.m.					
	6	7	8	9	10	11	12	1	2	3	4	5	6	7	8	9	10	11	12	1	2	3	4	5	6
Activities																									
Sleep Time																									

LIGHTS OUT_____ a.m. / p.m.   TOTAL SLEEP TIME_____ hrs

		p.m.						midnight / a.m.												noon / p.m.					
	6	7	8	9	10	11	12	1	2	3	4	5	6	7	8	9	10	11	12	1	2	3	4	5	6
Activities																									
Sleep Time																									

LIGHTS OUT_____ a.m. / p.m.   TOTAL SLEEP TIME_____ hrs

	p.m.							midnight / a.m.												noon / p.m.					
	6	7	8	9	10	11	12	1	2	3	4	5	6	7	8	9	10	11	12	1	2	3	4	5	6
Activities																									
Sleep Time																									

LIGHTS OUT_____ a.m. / p.m.   TOTAL SLEEP TIME_____ hrs

	p.m.							midnight / a.m.												noon / p.m.					
	6	7	8	9	10	11	12	1	2	3	4	5	6	7	8	9	10	11	12	1	2	3	4	5	6
Activities																									
Sleep Time																									

LIGHTS OUT_____ a.m. / p.m.   TOTAL SLEEP TIME_____ hrs

	p.m.							midnight / a.m.												noon / p.m.					
	6	7	8	9	10	11	12	1	2	3	4	5	6	7	8	9	10	11	12	1	2	3	4	5	6
Activities																									
Sleep Time																									

LIGHTS OUT_____ a.m. / p.m.   TOTAL SLEEP TIME_____ hrs

	p.m.							midnight / a.m.												noon / p.m.					
	6	7	8	9	10	11	12	1	2	3	4	5	6	7	8	9	10	11	12	1	2	3	4	5	6
Activities																									
Sleep Time																									

LIGHTS OUT_____ a.m. / p.m.   TOTAL SLEEP TIME_____ hrs

Week 2

	p.m.						midnight / a.m.												noon / p.m.						
	6	7	8	9	10	11	12	1	2	3	4	5	6	7	8	9	10	11	12	1	2	3	4	5	6
Activities																									
Sleep Time																									

LIGHTS OUT_____ a.m. / p.m.   TOTAL SLEEP TIME_____hrs

	p.m.						midnight / a.m.												noon / p.m.						
	6	7	8	9	10	11	12	1	2	3	4	5	6	7	8	9	10	11	12	1	2	3	4	5	6
Activities																									
Sleep Time																									

LIGHTS OUT_____ a.m. / p.m.   TOTAL SLEEP TIME_____hrs

	p.m.						midnight / a.m.												noon / p.m.						
	6	7	8	9	10	11	12	1	2	3	4	5	6	7	8	9	10	11	12	1	2	3	4	5	6
Activities																									
Sleep Time																									

LIGHTS OUT_____ a.m. / p.m.   TOTAL SLEEP TIME_____hrs

Chart 1

	p.m.						midnight / a.m.												noon / p.m.					
	6	7	8	9	10	11	12	1	2	3	4	5	6	7	8	9	10	11	12	1	2	3	4	5	6
Activities																									
Sleep Time																									

LIGHTS OUT_____ a.m. / p.m.   TOTAL SLEEP TIME_____ hrs

Chart 2

	p.m.						midnight / a.m.												noon / p.m.					
	6	7	8	9	10	11	12	1	2	3	4	5	6	7	8	9	10	11	12	1	2	3	4	5	6
Activities																									
Sleep Time																									

LIGHTS OUT_____ a.m. / p.m.   TOTAL SLEEP TIME_____ hrs

Chart 3

	p.m.						midnight / a.m.												noon / p.m.					
	6	7	8	9	10	11	12	1	2	3	4	5	6	7	8	9	10	11	12	1	2	3	4	5	6
Activities																									
Sleep Time																									

LIGHTS OUT_____ a.m. / p.m.   TOTAL SLEEP TIME_____ hrs

Chart 4

	p.m.						midnight / a.m.												noon / p.m.					
	6	7	8	9	10	11	12	1	2	3	4	5	6	7	8	9	10	11	12	1	2	3	4	5	6
Activities																									
Sleep Time																									

LIGHTS OUT_____ a.m. / p.m.   TOTAL SLEEP TIME_____ hrs

Week 3

	p.m.						midnight / a.m.												noon / p.m.					
	6	7	8	9	10	11	12	1	2	3	4	5	6	7	8	9	10	11	12	1	2	3	4	5	6
Activities																									
Sleep Time																									

LIGHTS OUT_____ a.m. / p.m.   TOTAL SLEEP TIME_____ hrs

	p.m.						midnight / a.m.												noon / p.m.					
	6	7	8	9	10	11	12	1	2	3	4	5	6	7	8	9	10	11	12	1	2	3	4	5	6
Activities																									
Sleep Time																									

LIGHTS OUT_____ a.m. / p.m.   TOTAL SLEEP TIME_____ hrs

	p.m.						midnight / a.m.												noon / p.m.					
	6	7	8	9	10	11	12	1	2	3	4	5	6	7	8	9	10	11	12	1	2	3	4	5	6
Activities																									
Sleep Time																									

LIGHTS OUT_____ a.m. / p.m.   TOTAL SLEEP TIME_____ hrs

Chart 1

	p.m.						midnight / a.m.																		noon / p.m.	
	6	7	8	9	10	11	12	1	2	3	4	5	6	7	8	9	10	11	12	1	2	3	4	5	6
Activities																									
Sleep Time																									

LIGHTS OUT_____ a.m. / p.m. TOTAL SLEEP TIME_____ hrs

Chart 2

	p.m.						midnight / a.m.																		noon / p.m.	
	6	7	8	9	10	11	12	1	2	3	4	5	6	7	8	9	10	11	12	1	2	3	4	5	6
Activities																									
Sleep Time																									

LIGHTS OUT_____ a.m. / p.m. TOTAL SLEEP TIME_____ hrs

Chart 3

	p.m.						midnight / a.m.																		noon / p.m.	
	6	7	8	9	10	11	12	1	2	3	4	5	6	7	8	9	10	11	12	1	2	3	4	5	6
Activities																									
Sleep Time																									

LIGHTS OUT_____ a.m. / p.m. TOTAL SLEEP TIME_____ hrs

Chart 4

	p.m.						midnight / a.m.																		noon / p.m.	
	6	7	8	9	10	11	12	1	2	3	4	5	6	7	8	9	10	11	12	1	2	3	4	5	6
Activities																									
Sleep Time																									

LIGHTS OUT_____ a.m. / p.m. TOTAL SLEEP TIME_____ hrs

Week 4

	p.m.						midnight / a.m.												noon / p.m.					
	6	7	8	9	10	11	12	1	2	3	4	5	6	7	8	9	10	11	12	1	2	3	4	5	6
Activities																									
Sleep Time																									

LIGHTS OUT_____ a.m. / p.m.   TOTAL SLEEP TIME_____hrs

	p.m.						midnight / a.m.												noon / p.m.					
	6	7	8	9	10	11	12	1	2	3	4	5	6	7	8	9	10	11	12	1	2	3	4	5	6
Activities																									
Sleep Time																									

LIGHTS OUT_____ a.m. / p.m.   TOTAL SLEEP TIME_____hrs

	p.m.						midnight / a.m.												noon / p.m.					
	6	7	8	9	10	11	12	1	2	3	4	5	6	7	8	9	10	11	12	1	2	3	4	5	6
Activities																									
Sleep Time																									

LIGHTS OUT_____ a.m. / p.m.   TOTAL SLEEP TIME_____hrs

	p.m.							midnight / a.m.												noon / p.m.					
	6	7	8	9	10	11	12	1	2	3	4	5	6	7	8	9	10	11	12	1	2	3	4	5	6
Activities																									
Sleep Time																									

LIGHTS OUT_____ a.m. / p.m.   TOTAL SLEEP TIME_____ hrs

	p.m.							midnight / a.m.												noon / p.m.					
	6	7	8	9	10	11	12	1	2	3	4	5	6	7	8	9	10	11	12	1	2	3	4	5	6
Activities																									
Sleep Time																									

LIGHTS OUT_____ a.m. / p.m.   TOTAL SLEEP TIME_____ hrs

	p.m.							midnight / a.m.												noon / p.m.					
	6	7	8	9	10	11	12	1	2	3	4	5	6	7	8	9	10	11	12	1	2	3	4	5	6
Activities																									
Sleep Time																									

LIGHTS OUT_____ a.m. / p.m.   TOTAL SLEEP TIME_____ hrs

	p.m.							midnight / a.m.												noon / p.m.					
	6	7	8	9	10	11	12	1	2	3	4	5	6	7	8	9	10	11	12	1	2	3	4	5	6
Activities																									
Sleep Time																									

LIGHTS OUT_____ a.m. / p.m.   TOTAL SLEEP TIME_____ hrs

Week 5

	p.m.					midnight / a.m.												noon / p.m.					
	6	7	8	9	10	11	12	1	2	3	4	5	6	7	8	9	10	11	12	1	2	3	4	5	6
Activities																									
Sleep Time																										

LIGHTS OUT_____ a.m. / p.m.   TOTAL SLEEP TIME_____ hrs

	p.m.					midnight / a.m.												noon / p.m.					
	6	7	8	9	10	11	12	1	2	3	4	5	6	7	8	9	10	11	12	1	2	3	4	5	6
Activities																										
Sleep Time																										

LIGHTS OUT_____ a.m. / p.m.   TOTAL SLEEP TIME_____ hrs

	p.m.					midnight / a.m.												noon / p.m.					
	6	7	8	9	10	11	12	1	2	3	4	5	6	7	8	9	10	11	12	1	2	3	4	5	6
Activities																										
Sleep Time																										

LIGHTS OUT_____ a.m. / p.m.   TOTAL SLEEP TIME_____ hrs

Sleep log (blank chart, repeated four times).

Chart 1

	p.m.						midnight / a.m.												noon / p.m.			
	6	7	8	9	10	11	12	1	2	3	4	5	6	7	8	9	10	11	12	1	2	3	4	5	6
Activities																									
Sleep Time																									

LIGHTS OUT_____ a.m. / p.m.   TOTAL SLEEP TIME_____ hrs

Chart 2

	p.m.						midnight / a.m.												noon / p.m.			
	6	7	8	9	10	11	12	1	2	3	4	5	6	7	8	9	10	11	12	1	2	3	4	5	6
Activities																									
Sleep Time																									

LIGHTS OUT_____ a.m. / p.m.   TOTAL SLEEP TIME_____ hrs

Chart 3

	p.m.						midnight / a.m.												noon / p.m.			
	6	7	8	9	10	11	12	1	2	3	4	5	6	7	8	9	10	11	12	1	2	3	4	5	6
Activities																									
Sleep Time																									

LIGHTS OUT_____ a.m. / p.m.   TOTAL SLEEP TIME_____ hrs

Chart 4

	p.m.						midnight / a.m.												noon / p.m.			
	6	7	8	9	10	11	12	1	2	3	4	5	6	7	8	9	10	11	12	1	2	3	4	5	6
Activities																									
Sleep Time																									

LIGHTS OUT_____ a.m. / p.m.   TOTAL SLEEP TIME_____ hrs

Week 6

	p.m.						midnight / a.m.												noon / p.m.						
	6	7	8	9	10	11	12	1	2	3	4	5	6	7	8	9	10	11	12	1	2	3	4	5	6
Activities																									
Sleep Time																									

LIGHTS OUT_____ a.m. / p.m.   TOTAL SLEEP TIME_____ hrs

	p.m.						midnight / a.m.												noon / p.m.						
	6	7	8	9	10	11	12	1	2	3	4	5	6	7	8	9	10	11	12	1	2	3	4	5	6
Activities																									
Sleep Time																									

LIGHTS OUT_____ a.m. / p.m.   TOTAL SLEEP TIME_____ hrs

	p.m.						midnight / a.m.												noon / p.m.						
	6	7	8	9	10	11	12	1	2	3	4	5	6	7	8	9	10	11	12	1	2	3	4	5	6
Activities																									
Sleep Time																									

LIGHTS OUT_____ a.m. / p.m.   TOTAL SLEEP TIME_____ hrs

	p.m.							midnight / a.m.												noon / p.m.					
	6	7	8	9	10	11	12	1	2	3	4	5	6	7	8	9	10	11	12	1	2	3	4	5	6
Activities																									
Sleep Time																									

LIGHTS OUT_____ a.m. / p.m.   TOTAL SLEEP TIME_____ hrs

	6	7	8	9	10	11	12	1	2	3	4	5	6	7	8	9	10	11	12	1	2	3	4	5	6
Activities																									
Sleep Time																									

LIGHTS OUT_____ a.m. / p.m.   TOTAL SLEEP TIME_____ hrs

	6	7	8	9	10	11	12	1	2	3	4	5	6	7	8	9	10	11	12	1	2	3	4	5	6
Activities																									
Sleep Time																									

LIGHTS OUT_____ a.m. / p.m.   TOTAL SLEEP TIME_____ hrs

	6	7	8	9	10	11	12	1	2	3	4	5	6	7	8	9	10	11	12	1	2	3	4	5	6
Activities																									
Sleep Time																									

LIGHTS OUT_____ a.m. / p.m.   TOTAL SLEEP TIME_____ hrs

Progressive muscle relaxation

You will tense each muscle group vigorously, but without straining, and then suddenly release the tension and feel the muscle relax. You will tense each muscle for about five seconds. If you have any pain or discomfort at any of the targeted muscle groups, feel free to omit that step. Throughout this exercise try to visualise the muscles tensing and a wave of relaxation flowing over them as you release that tension. It is important that you keep breathing throughout the exercise. Now let's begin. . .

Start by finding a comfortable position either sitting or lying down in a location where you will not be interrupted.

Allow your attention to focus only on your body. If you begin to notice your mind wandering, bring it back to the muscle you are working on.

Take a deep breath through your abdomen, hold for a few seconds and exhale slowly. As you breathe notice your stomach rising and your lungs filling with air. As you exhale, imagine the tension in your body being released and flowing out of your body. And again inhale . . . and exhale. Feel your body already relaxing. As you go through each step, remember to keep breathing.

Now let's begin going through the muscles. Tighten the muscles in your forehead by raising your eyebrows as high as you can. Hold for about five seconds. And abruptly release, feeling that tension fall away.

Pause for about ten seconds.

Now smile widely, feeling your mouth and cheeks tense. Hold for about five seconds and release, appreciating the softness in your face. Pause for about ten seconds.

Next, tense your eye muscles by squeezing your eyelids tightly shut. Hold for about five seconds and release. Pause for about ten seconds.

Gently pull your head back as if to look at the ceiling. Hold for about five seconds, and release, feeling the tension melting away. Pause for about ten seconds. Now feel the weight of your relaxed head and neck sink. Breathe in . . . and out. In . . . and out. Let go of all the stress. In . . . and out.

Now, tightly, but without straining, clench your fists and hold this position for about five seconds, and then release. Pause for about ten seconds.

Now, flex your biceps. Feel that build-up of tension. You may even visualise the muscle tightening. Hold for about five seconds and release, enjoying that feeling of limpness. Breathe in . . . and out.

Now tighten your triceps by extending your arms out and locking your elbows. Hold for about five seconds and release. Pause for about ten seconds.

Now lift your shoulders up as if they could touch your ears. Hold for about five seconds and quickly release, feeling their heaviness. Pause for about ten seconds.

Tense your upper back by pulling your shoulders back, trying to make your shoulder blades touch. Hold for about five seconds and release. Pause for about ten seconds.

Tighten your chest by taking a deep breath in, hold for about five seconds and exhale, blowing out all the tension.

Now tighten the muscles in your stomach by sucking in. Hold for about five seconds and release. Pause for about ten seconds.

Gently arch your lower back. Hold for about five seconds, relax. Pause for about ten seconds.

Feel the limpness in your upper body letting go of the tension and stress. Pause for about five seconds and relax.

Tighten your buttocks. Hold for about five seconds ... and release, imagine your hips falling loose. Pause for about ten seconds.

Tighten your thighs by pressing your knees together, as if you were holding a penny between them. Hold for about five seconds . . . and release. Pause for about ten seconds.

Now flex your feet, pulling your toes towards you and feeling the tension in your calves. Hold for about five seconds and relax. Feel the weight of your legs sinking down. Pause for about ten seconds.

Curl your toes under, tensing your feet. Hold for about five seconds, release. Pause for about ten seconds.

Now imagine a wave of relaxation slowly spreading through your body beginning at your head and going all the way down to your feet. Feel the weight of your relaxed body. Breathe in . . . and out. In . . . out. In . . . out.

If you would like an audiofile that you can download, this is one helpful example from the Northumbria Tyne and Wear NHS trust.

www.ntw.nhs.uk/content/uploads/2017/06/F_06_
Progressive-Muscle-Relaxation.mp3

Further information about obstructive sleep apnoea

This can be found on the British Lung Foundation website, which has detailed information about obstructive sleep apnoea (OSA) including diagnosis, investigations and treatment. www.blf.org.uk/support-for-you/osa

Epworth sleepiness score

This is a simple self-rated list of eight questions to measure how sleepy you feel during the day. The Epworth can be found on the website of the British Lung Foundation, www.blf.org.uk/support-for-you/obstructive-sleep-apnoea-osa/diagnosis/epworth-sleepiness-scale and refers to how likely you are to actually doze or snooze rather than feel fatigued and asks you to think about the last month when you are filling in the questions. Most of us will feel sleepy sometimes and so the normal ranges for the adult population are between 4 and 10. Those who really struggle to fall asleep and have insomnia are more likely to have scores that are lower than normal at 0, 1 or 2. Scores that are over 10 are more common with other sleep problems.

The NHS has lots of good information about treatment for sleep and insomnia as well as other sleep disorders and this can be found at www.nhs.uk/conditions/insomnia

More information about exercise

If you haven't done exercise for some time, then it might be a good idea to read a little more about different types of exercise and what is meant by moderate or high intensity. There are some helpful links below which can help you to get started with a whole range of activities.

It really doesn't matter what type of exercise you do as long as you are doing something but check with your GP if you have concerns about any other medical conditions that you think might stop you doing a particular activity.

www.nhs.uk/Livewell/fitness/Pages/physical-activity-guidelines-for-adults.aspx

www.nhs.uk/Livewell/getting-started-guides/Pages/getting-started-guides.aspx

INDEX

Notes

1. The word order is word-by-word; and
2. Locators of forms and tables are in *italics*.

A

Advanced Sleep Phase
    Syndrome 53
alcohol 69–70
Auton, Rob 34
awake in bed 74, 83–4

B

bad sleepers 38
bedrooms 71–4
beds 82–5
bedtimes 86–8
biological (body) clock *see*
    circadian rhythms
brain activity 22, 33
Brontë, Charlotte 98

C

caffeine 66–9
Carlin, George 21

CBT for insomnia (CBTi)
    3, 4
children 37
circadian rhythms 23–7,
    36, 52–3, 113
clocks 73
Cognitive Behavioural
    Therapy (CBT) 1–2
cognitive control
    techniques 100–5
comorbid insomnia 42
concentration 26, 35

D

darkness 72
daytime activities 85
Delayed Sleep Phase
    Syndrome 53
depression 35
dream sleep (REM sleep)
    33

E
Epworth sleepiness score
    164
exercise 70–1, 107, 165

F
family and friends 13
feeling wide awake 83–5,
    96, 97, 108, 113–14

G
getting up in the night 84
goals 15, *16–19*
good and bad days 11–12
good sleepers 38
GPs 12–13

H
homeostat 22–3, 25–6,
    90, 113

I
Improving Access
    to Psychological
    Therapies (IAPT) 14
insomnia 38–41

L
laptops 73, 85
lifestyle factors 75–6, *77*
light/light sources 25, 72, 74

M
memory 35
mental health 35, 42
motivation to change
    14–16
muscle tension 103–4

N
narcolepsy 54–5
nicotine 70
night owls 36
night-time waking 34
nightmares 53–4
noise 72
non-dream sleep (NREM
    sleep) 33
normal sleep *33*, 36
number techniques 102–3

O
obstructive sleep apnoea
    (OSA) 51–2, 164

P
parasomnias 53–4
Paul (case study) 30–3, 74,
    139–43
persistent insomnia 39–41
phones 73, 85
Poppy (case study) 27–9,
    40, 115–38
    sleep diary 80–1, 90,
        94–5
    sleep efficiency 78–9,
        85–6, 127, 132
professional support 14
progressive muscle
    relaxation 103–4,
    160–3
Psychological Wellbeing
    Practitioners (PWPs)
    14

Q
quarter-hour rule 84–5

R

racing minds 97, 100–5
relapse prevention toolkit
    105–9
relaxation 75, 103–4
REM sleep (dream sleep)
    33
restless legs syndrome
    (RLS) 49–50

S

'*schlafzimmer*' ('sleep
    room') 74, 114
sex 85
short sleepers 36
sleep
    and beds 82–5
    how much we need
        35–7
    importance 34–5
    stages 33
sleep diary 15–16, 58–65,
    106, 112, 145–59
sleep disorders 48–55
sleep efficiency 79, 85–6,
    91–2
sleep hygiene 65–6, 76
sleep paralysis 54–5
sleep patterns 37, 62,
    76–8, 86–90
sleep restriction 78, 82,
    85–92
sleep scheduling 76–82,
    90–6
sleep time 78–9

sleep-wake cycle 25, 107
sleeping rules 88–9
sleeping tablets 42–8
sleepwalking 53–4
sleepy at bedtime 82,
    84–5, 108, 113
smoking 70
snoring 51–2
stimulus control 78, 82
suprachiasmatic nucleus
    (SCN) 25

T

teenagers 37
thinking about sleep 41
time in bed (TIB) 78–9
'tossing and turning'
    103–4
total sleep time (TST)
    78–9
TVs 74, 85

U

unwanted behaviours
    53–4

V

verbal techniques 102
visualisation techniques
    101

W

waking times 86
winding-down 75–6, 98–9
work-related activities 75